SOCIAL AND MEDICAL ASPECTS OF DRUG ABUSE

edited by
George Serban, M.D.
Principal Research Investigator
and Clinical Associate Professor
Department of Psychiatry
New York University School of Medicine
New York, New York

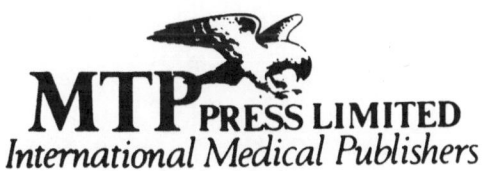

MTP PRESS LIMITED
International Medical Publishers

Published in the UK and Europe by
MTP Press Limited
Falcon House
Lancaster, England

Published in the US by
SPECTRUM PUBLICATIONS, INC.
175-20 Wexford Terrace
Jamaica, NY 11432

ISBN-13: 978-94-011-6322-4   e-ISBN-13: 978-94-011-6320-0
DOI: 10.1007/ 978-94-011-6320-0

Contributors

Paul Cushman, Jr., M.D. • Associate Professor of Medicine and Psychiatry, De Paul Rehabilitation Hospital, Milwaukee, Wisconsin

Judianne Densen-Gerber, M.D. • President, Odyssey Institute International, New York, New York

Don C. Des Jarlais, Ph.D. • Assistant Deputy Director for Substance Abuse Research and Evaluation, Division of Substance Abuse Services, New York, New York

P. B. Dews, M.D. • Professor of Psychiatry, Laboratory of Psychobiology, Harvard Medical School, Boston, Massachusetts

Blanche Frank, Ph.D. • Chief of Epidemiology, State of New York Division of Substance Abuse Services, Office of Alcoholism and Substance Abuse, New York, New York

Harold M. Ginzburg, M.D. • Chief, Clinical Behavioral Branch, Division of Research, NIDA, Rockville, Maryland

Leif Gronbladh, M.D. • Uppsala University, Uppsala, Sweden

Robert Greenstein, M.D. • Veterans Administration Outpatient Clinic, Philadelphia, Pennsylvania

Lars M. Gunne, M.D. • Head of Psychiatric Research Center, Professor of Psychiatry, Ulleraker Hospital, Uppsala, Sweden

Bruce J. Johnson, Ph.D. • Director of the Interdisciplinary Research Center, State of New York Division of Substance Abuse Services, Office of Alcoholism and Substance Abuse, New York, New York

Herbert D. Kleber, M.D. • Professor of Psychiatry; Director, Substance Abuse Treatment Unit, Addiction Prevention, Treatment Foundation, Yale University School of Medicine, Department of Psychiatry, New Haven, Connecticut

Douglas S. Lipton, Ph.D. • State of New York Division of Substance Abuse Services, Office of Alcoholism and Substance Abuse, New York, New York

Robert A. Markowitz, Ph.D. • Research Pharmacologist, Clinical Behavioral Branch, NIDA, Rockville, Maryland

William R. Martin, M.D. • Professor and Chairman, Department of Pharmacology, University of Kentucky, Lexington, Kentucky

Steven M. Mirin, M.D. • Associate Professor of Psychiatry, Harvard Medical School, Boston; Director, Drug Dependence Treatment Unit, McLean Hospital, Belmont, Massachusetts

S. Joseph Mulé, Ph.D. • Director, State of New York Division of Substance Abuse Services, Testing and Research Laboratories; Professor of Psychiatry, State University of New York, Downstate Medical Center, Brooklyn, New York

William Pollin, M.D. • Director, Division of Research, NIDA, Rockville, Maryland

Charles P. O'Brien, M.D., Ph.D. • Professor of Psychiatry; Chief, Psychiatry Services; Director, Drug Treatment and Research Center, Veterans Administration Medical Center, Philadelphia, Pennsylvania

Richard B. Resnick, M.D. • Department of Psychiatry, New York Medical College, Valhalla, New York

Bruce J. Rounsaville, M.D. • Assistant Professor of Psychiatry, Yale University School of Medicine, New Haven, Connecticut

George Serban, M.D. • Research Psychiatrist; Clinical Associate Professor, Department of Psychiatry, New York University School of Medicine, New York, New York

Eric J. Simon, Ph.D. • Professor of Psychiatry and Pharmacology, New York University School of Medicine, New York, New York

Ian P. Stolerman, Ph.D. • Honorary Senior Lecturer, Department of Pharmacology, Institute of Psychiatry, De Crespigny Park, London, England

Joseph W. Ternes, Ph.D. • Veterans Administration Medical Center, Philadelphia, Pennsylvania

Karl Verebey, Ph.D. • Director of Clinical Pharmacology, Testing and Research Laboratory; Associate Professor, New York State Division of Substance Abuse, State University of New York, Downstate Medical School, Brooklyn, New York

Arnold M. Washton, Ph.D. • Department of Psychiatry, New York Medical College, Valhalla, New York

Myrna M. Weissman, M.D. • Professor of Research, Department of Psychiatry, Yale University School of Medicine, New Haven, Connecticut

Charles H. Wilbur, M.D. • Department of Psychiatry, Yale University School of Medicine, New Haven, Connecticut

George E. Woody, M.D. • Chief, Drug Dependence Treatment Unit, Veterans Administration Medical Center, Philadelphia, Pennsylvania

R. Suzanne Zukin, Ph.D. • Assistant Professor, Department of Biochemistry and Neuroscience, Albert Einstein College of Medicine of Yeshiva University, New York, New York

Steven R. Zukin, M.D. • Departments of Biochemistry and Neuroscience, Albert Einstein College of Medicine of Yeshiva University, New York, New York

Foreword

The phenomenon of drug abuse is part of the human experience that extends as far back in time as recorded history exists. Today, however, it has a new and much greater dramatic urgency. The reasons for this are multiple and worrisome. Last year, of the total of approximately 1.9 million total deaths that occurred in the United States, a conservative estimate is that more than one-quarter were premature deaths due to the addictive disorders. These include over 300,000 deaths related to cigarette smoking, which represents in many respects the prototypic addiction in this country; over 200,000 deaths related to alcohol, and many more related to multiple other drugs—licit and illicit—that are abused in this society.

Twenty-five years ago, drug use was essentially unknown in our school age population. In 1960, a tragic increase of drug use in our young people began, so that by 1978 more high school seniors were current users of marijuana than of cigarettes. Despite the fact that the use of most drugs by high school populations appears to have peaked in the late 1970s and to be decreasing at the present time, most experts still believe that drug use by American young people represents the highest level of that found in any Western developed country.

There are important demographic changes taking place in the United States which suggest that during the next fifteen years, the level use of drugs in this country may decrease. On the other hand, at the same time, we are in the midst of a period of even more rapid discovery of increasingly powerful psychoactive drugs. Each such discovery, given the increasing technical proficiency which simplifies their production, increases the number of substances which will likely be abused in the future; thus, the potential dimensions of this problem are, in many respects, on a growth curve.

There has been an explosive increase not only in the dimensions and complexity of the problem of drug use and abuse in this country and in the world during the past two decades, but, in parallel, an explosive increase in our knowledge concerning these phenomena. For the first time, we have begun to understand the biology of behavior and, as great strides have been made in the study of brain/behavior relationships, we find that many of the drugs which are most subject to abuse and involved in addictive behaviors are drugs that play a key role in the biology of affect and reinforcement. Thus, for example, the discovery of the body's own morphine-like compounds—the endorphins and the enkephalins—have led for the first time to the development of eventually testable hypotheses which define a biological set of mechanisms, related to reward and reinforcement systems, that can explain narcotic addiction. Some investigators have suggested that disorders in the production, metabolism, or receptor sensitivity to endorphins may, in a pattern not unlike the body's handling of insulin in diabetes, be one of the factors that contributes to increased vulnerability to narcotic addiction among certain individuals or subpopulations. I am not suggesting here that this is likely to be demonstrated; I merely use it as an example of a new kind of hypothesis, testable eventually by empiric data, which was not available to us a decade ago.

The National Institute on Drug Abuse is proud of the key role it played in helping to encourage and support a wide range of basic biological, social, and psychobehavioral research, many of the fruits of which are reflected in the following chapters. The Institute looks forward to playing a similar role in the future. We anticipate further and accelerated advances in the areas of knowledge development and knowledge application, to the end of understanding and helping society to control and ameliorate the major problems associated with drug abuse in the twentieth century.

William Pollin, M.D.
Director, National Institute
on Drug Abuse

Preface

Though from the medical point of view the problem of addiction appears to be limited in scope and dearth, its implication for society is vast. The use of drugs is responsible for the lack of safety in the community, violence on the streets, increase in the price of goods due to loss of billions in shoplifting, and reduction in productivity. In one study reported by a Philadelphia group, each addict of this group of 237 committed about 192 crimes yearly.

The acuteness of the drug problem is reflected in the continuous increase in the use of drugs by the high school population. Thirty-seven percent of the seniors in high school are marijuana users and 11% use it daily. One and a half million teenagers between 12 and 17 have used PCP. This is an increase of 50% over 1976 statistics. In addition, 4.2 million young adults between 18 and 25 are experimenting with PCP, while 21% of the age group 12-25 have used amphetamines. The young population, compared to the adult population, shows a higher rate of use of all types of drugs.

This alarming spread of drugs is not being checked by comparable means of treatment and prevention. Our knowledge about the prevention and method of treatment appears to be insufficient to cope with the abuse of drugs, which has become almost impossible to contain. All research related to either treatment or prevention has proved to be inconclusive.

Our knowledge about the abuse of drugs is fragmented and contradictory. Our approach to it lacks consistency. If we have been successful in treating the problem of withdrawal medically, we have failed utterly in maintaining the ex-addict free of drugs in the community. Eighty percent of all heroin abusers are relapsing within 12 months of the termination of treatment. The problem of drug addiction surpasses the medical perimeters of concern and projects itself into the very essence of the societal conflicts of our time.

It is a part of a pervasive social sickness. Society has become highly hedonistic, drug oriented, and non-achievement directed (until recently). The drug problem can be partially prevented by control of the smuggling of drugs, or by better and more creative means of educating the public. Its true elimination depends on a reevaluation of our social aims and aspirations and redefinitions of the values and meaning of life for the individual. It is a fact that our tolerant approach to deviant behavior, be it criminal or drug abuse, didn't work out well for society. In general, the socially deviant did not become more socially integrated, less violent, or less hedonistically oriented by our permissiveness. On the contrary, they abused permissiveness, using it for their own deviant needs and self gratification. The leniency toward crime resulting from drug addiction, the emphasis of the medical model that drug addiction is only a mental and physical illness and not also a social problem, promoted indirectly the abuse of drugs by making the individual feel not responsible for his actions.

This book attempts to define a new approach to drug addiction based on a biopsychosocial model in which all the components of human interaction with the environment are integrated and attacked simultaneously. The individual has to feel that society will help him solve his problems but will not carry him on his hedonistic terms because he labelled himself as such and acts out as a drug user.

We believe the book will stimulate new approaches, while evaluating the efficacy of the present one, with the result of pushing forward our knowledge in this complex field.

GEORGE SERBAN, M.D.
Medical Director
International Anti-Drug Abuse Foundation
New York, New York

ACKNOWLEDGMENTS

The international symposium "Drug Abuse: Social and Medical Issues," upon which this book is based, was sponsored by the International Anti-Drug Abuse Foundation, and held on April 27-29, 1981, at Vista International Hotel, World Trade Center, through the courtesy of Mr. Eddy J.M. Florijn, General Manager.

Special thanks are due also to Aviva Najar, International Chairman of the International Anti-Drug Abuse Foundation, and L. Howard Samuels, New York Chairman.

Contents

1

Relationship of Biological Influences on the Subjective States of Addicts

WILLIAM R. MARTIN

Drug abuse is a complex disease with complex dimensions. The epidemiologists have shown that many, not all, drug abusers come from disadvantaged environments. The psychiatrists and psychologists have long recognized that addicts have pathologic personality characteristics. Haertzen (1978) has recently reviewed a large body of data concerning the MMPI profiles of drug abusers. It is clear that all types of drug abusers including narcotic addicts, alcoholics, and poly-drug abusers have elevated scores on the Psychopathic Deviate (Pd) and the Depression (D) scales. Many addicts also have elevated scores on the Schizophrenia (Sc) and Hypomania (Ma) scale. On the basis of this psychologic testing, therefore, the addict appears to have a diffuse psychopathology. However, addicts seem to be remarkably normal; they have a normal range of intelligence, they show no consistent medical pathologies, and most are not psychotic. What then is their pathology?

> Their pathology in a large part is characterized by unfulfilled expectations. To political leaders and administrators this is a failure to realize their potential as tax payers; to their neighbors a failure to contribute meaningfully to their communities; to the consumer a failure to be sufficiently productive. The failure of the addict to fulfill social expectations in a society becoming increasingly characterized by mutual dependencies is their pathology (Martin, 1977).

The abuses of drugs are cardinal signs of sociopathic behavior. The phenomenon of drug abuse has helped in defining the role of drugs in this

1

destructive subtle psychopathology that has such profound social implications. I would like to review briefly efforts in which I participated over a period of almost twenty years that attempted to define the role of drug use in the pathology of drug abuse and to define the subjective effects of abused drugs that were responsible for their reinforcing effects.

Harris Hill and his collaborators (Hill et al, 1963) devised the Addiction Research Center Inventory (ARCI), a 500-item questionnaire containing many questions useful in measuring and conceptualizing subjective effects of drugs. One of the scales of particular importance which was derived from the ARCI was the MBG (morphine benzadrine group) scale. This scale measures feelings of enhanced self image, efficiency, and popularity. In an attempt to validate this scale, as well as other scales and questionnaires, a number of drugs were studied including a variety of narcotic analgesics, agonists-antagonists, amphetamines, and barbiturates. All of these abused drugs produced a dose related increase in the scale scores of the MBG scale. These observations were important for two reasons: (1) The observation that feelings of improved self-image, efficiency, and popularity were changed in a dose related manner suggested that they had an organic neuronal basis. (2) There is every reason to believe that these diverse drugs exert their effects through different modes of action, a point which is discussed later. Thus, the brain appears to have multiple neurohumoral processes that are involved in feelings of well being.

The next series of experiments that I would like to turn to were related to the process of physical dependence. The clarification of the concept of physical dependence and the identification of its characteristics were major advances in the study of the addiction process. Drugs such as the narcotic analgesics, barbiturates, and alcohol produce a type of physical dependence characterized by an explosive early abstinent syndrome. Although Himmelsbach (1942) had obtained evidence suggesting that the morphine abstinence syndrome might be prolonged, the first definitive demonstration of a protracted abstinence syndrome was done in rats by Dr. Wikler and myself. In experiments conducted to characterizing the time course of the morphine abstinent syndrome (Martin et al, 1963), the early abstinent syndrome in the rat ran its time course in about three days, and thereafter another abstinent syndrome emerged which had characteristics different from the early abstinent syndrome. This abstinent syndrome persisted and was still present in a diminished form 180 days after the animals had been withdrawn. It was called secondary or protracted abstinence.

These studies were subsequently extended to the dog (Martin et al, 1974) and to man (Martin and Jasinski, 1969; Martin et al, 1973). In the study of Martin and Jasinski (1969) patients were admitted to the wards of the Addiction Research Center and had an opportunity to accommodate to the environment; control observations were made three times daily for a period of seven weeks. Patients were then given morphine chronically; the dose was escalated over a five-week period until they were stabilized at 240 mg/day. They remained at this dose level for 29 weeks following which they were withdrawn gradually over a three-week period. During the period of addiction the patients temperature was significantly increased ($0.3°C$), pupils constricted, and respiratory rate depressed. Following withdrawal, blood pressure, body temperature, and respiratory rate were significantly increased and pupils dilated. This syndrome persisted for about one month following complete withdrawal of the drug. Thereafter, another persisting abstinent syndrome was observed characterized by a significant decrease in blood pressure and body temperature with a marginally significant decrease in pulse rate and constriction of pupils ($p < 0.1$). This syndrome persisted through the 31st week of abstinence at which time the study was terminated.

An analysis of variance was done on these data which segregated out the between subjects, between weeks and between treatments variance. Although changes in blood pressure, temperature, and pulse rate were statistically significant, it was also found that the between subjects variance was only several times less than that of the treatment effects. This indicated that the characteristics of protracted abstinence syndrome fell within the range of normal values for the variables identified and that it would be probably impossible to diagnose protracted abstinence in an individual using these signs.

Observations were then extended to determine if protracted abstinence could also be observed following methadone withdrawal and to see if the physiologic changes were associated with changes in mood or feeling states (Martin et al, 1973). There was a protracted methadone abstinence syndrome in which blood pressure and body temperature were significantly less than control levels. Further, the methadone dependent patient in protracted abstinence showed an increase propensity to sleep and exhibited a variety of changes in mood that was characterized by elevated scale scores that indicated negative feeling states and a decrease in scores on scales that indicated positive feeling states. The ARCI and MMPI scales scores which were altered during the cycle of methadone dependence are summarized in Table 1. Thus the protracted abstinence syndrome is associated with feeling states that are opposite in polarity to the euphorigenic actions of the narcotic analgesics, sedative-hypnotics, and amphetamine-like drugs.

The feeling state present in protracted abstinence had some of the characteristics of depression but differed in some respects. Table 2 defines and compares euphoria, hypophoria, and depression. With regard to self-image the euphoric state is polarly opposite to hypophoria except in the estimation of self worth. Hypophoric patients feel they are worthy and deserving even though they are unappreciated. In contrast a high percentage of depressed

Table 1. ARCI Scales Which Are Significantly Changed
During Different Phases of the Addiction Cycle

Addiction	Early abstinence	Protracted abstinence
	Negative feelings increased	
PCAG	PCAG	Tiredness
Tiredness	Tiredness	Criticalness
	Social withdrawal	
	Criticalness	
	Positive feelings decreased	
Popularity	MBG	MBG
Efficiency	Efficiency	Popularity
	Competitiveness	Efficiency
	MMPI Scales elevated	
Hysteria	Hysteria	Schizophrenia
Hypochondriasis	Hypochondriasis	
Schizophrenia	Schizophrenia	

PCAG = Pentobarbital-Chlorpromazine-Alcohol Group Scale
MBG = Morphine-Benzadrine Group Scale

Table 2. Clinical Characteristics of Feelings Prevalent in the Mood States
Euphoria, Hypophoria and Depression

Euphoria (Feelings of well being)	Hypophoria	Depression
	Self image	
Popular	Unpopular	
Competent	Inept	
Efficient	Inefficient	
Appreciated	Unappreciated	
Worthy	Worthy	Worthless
	Outlook	
Hopeful	Hopeful	Hopeless
	Affect	
Can experience joy	Can experience joy	Cannot experience joy
Can laugh	Can laugh	Cannot laugh
	Guiltless	Guilty

patients feel unworthy (Woodruff et al, 1967). By and large hypophoric patients feel hopeful, can experience joy, enjoy humor, and laugh readily. In contrast, hopelessness and sadness are among the most common symptoms of depressed patients. Another important difference between the hypophoric and the depressed patient is the lack of guilt feelings in the hypophoric patient.

Analysis of the characteristics of sociopathy led us to identify five major traits: impulsivity, egocentricity, increased need states, feelings of hypophoria, and feelings related to sociopathic impulses. We constructed a questionnaire called the Maturation Scale. It was composed of five subscales which we felt measured existing feelings related to these five traits (Martin et al, 1977). We compared 53 students and teachers at a theologic seminary with 53 subjects who had been treated for alcoholism and 24 prisoners who were narcotic addicts. These subjects completed the Maturation Scale questionnaire, the MMPI, and an indepth Personal History Questionnaire which identified a number of types of sociopathic behavior. A partial content of the Personal History Questionnaire is presented in Table 3 (Hewett et al, 1980). The personal history questionnaire was constructed and scored such that it gave a quantitative estimate of the amount of sociopathic behavior that the subject had been involved in. The results obtained with the Maturation Scale, MMPI, and the Personal History Questionnaire for the three groups of subjects are presented in Table 4. Clearly both the alcoholics and the addicts had significant elevations on all of the subscales of the Maturation Scale, the Pd, Ma and D scale of the MMPI and the Adult Sociopathy Scale of the Personal History Questionnaire (Martin, 1977). These findings on the

Table 3. Personal History Content

1. Drug use and dependence	3. Developmental difficulties
	Learning problems
2. Sociopathic behavior	Daytime restlessness
Stealing	Sleep disorders
Fighting	Psychiatric problems
Dishonorable discharge	Pre-adult sociopathy
Arrests	Truancy
Imprisonments	Loss of parental control
Drug sales	Setting fires
Use of aliases	Fighting
Work instability	Stealing
Economic dependency	

Table 4. Maturation, MMPI, and Adult Sociopathy Scale Scores
(Mean ± SE)

	Controls (53)	Alcoholics (53)	Addict prisoners (24)
Impulsivity	0.3 ± 0.1	1.4* ± 0.2	1.2* ± 0.2
Egocentricity	1.2 ± 0.1	1.9* ± 0.2	1.5 ± 0.2
Need	3.0 ± 0.2	4.1* ± 0.2	5.0* ± 0.2
Sociopathy	2.3 ± 0.2	4.0* ± 0.3	6.3* ± 0.4
Hypophoria	6.9 ± 0.3	8.6* ± 0.5	11.0* ± 0.7
Maturation	13.6 ± 0.5	20.0* ± 0.9	24.8* ± 1.1
Pd	58 ± 1.4	73* ± 1.7	74* ± 1.7
Ma	54 ± 1.2	66* ± 1.6	70* ± 2.6
D	50 ± 1.0	65* ± 2.1	66* ± 2.9
Adult sociopathy scores	2.5 ± 0.4	25.2* ± 2.21	52.4* ± 3.4

*$p < 0.01$ comparison with controls

MMPI are in keeping with data obtained by others. The questions of the Maturation Scale asked the patients how they felt at the time they were completing the questionnaires and the Maturation Scale was devoid of any retrospective questions. The data obtained on these scales were correlated with Adult Sociopathy Scores from the Personal History Questionnaire. All of the subscales of the Maturation Scale and the Pd scale of the MMPI were significantly correlated with the scores on the Adult Sociopathy Scores (Martin, 1978). These data would indicate that, indeed, alcoholics and narcotic addicts do have an affective disorder and that this disorder of feelings is associated with antisocial behavior.

Hypophoria has the dimensions of feelings of lack of efficiency and popularity and a poor self image. As indicated above narcotic analgesics, amphetamines and barbiturates enhance feelings of well being and diminish feelings related to poor self image, inefficiency and unpopularity. In addition other drugs of abuse including marihuana and LSD-like hallucinogens also produce similar feelings of well being.

Feeling states may be under the control of proven neurohumors for we know that the narcotic analgesics share many features in common with brain peptides, the enkephalins and endorphins, that amphetamines release dopamine, that the LSD-like hallucinogens mimic the effects of tryptamine and serotonin both of which are endogenous brain transmitters and the barbiturate prolonged the action of the inhibitory transmitter GABA. One can speculate that patients with hypophoria may have a deficiency in one or more of these neurotransmitters involved in feeling states and that their personality disorder could have an organic basis. With the rapid development of the neurosciences it seems well within the realm of possibility that these deficiency states can be identified and diagnosed and that new drugs can be designed and developed which would rectify these disorders. Therefore, various types of antisocial behavior including drug abuse, which has been viewed from the point of view of ethical and a legal perspective, may indeed prove to be mental health disorders amenable to specific chemotherapy.

REFERENCES

Hewett BB and Martin WR: Psychometric comparisons of sociopathic and psycho-pathological behaviors of alcoholics and drug abusers versus a low drug use control population. *Int J Addict* 15:77-105, 1980

Hill HE, Haertzen CA, Wolbach HB and Miner EJ: The addiction research center inventory: Standardization of scales which evaluate subjective effects of morphine, amphetamine, pentobarbital, alcohol, LSD-25, pyrahexyl and chlorpromazine. *Psychopharmacologia* 4:167-183, 1963

Himmelsbach CK: Clinical studies of drug addiction; physical dependence withdrawal and recovery. *Arch Intern Med* 69:776-782, 1942

Martin WR: Drugs and drug addiction. Pg. 1-11 Proceedings of the 39th Annual Scientific Meeting of the Committee on Problems of Drug Dependence, 1977

Martin WR, Hewett BB, Baker AJ and Haertzen CA: Aspects of the psychopathology and pathophysiology of addiction. *Drug Alc Depend* 2:185-202, 1977

Martin WR and Jasinski DR: Physiological parameters of morphine dependence in man—tolerance, early abstinence, protracted abstinence. *J Psychiat Res* 7:9-17, 1969

Martin WR, Jasinski DR, Haertzen CA, Kay DC, Jones BE, Mansky PA and Carpenter RW: Methadone—A reevaluation. *Arch Gen Psychiatr* 28:286-295, 1973

Martin WR, Wikler A, Eades CG and Prescor FT: Tolerance to and physical dependence on morphine in rats. *Psychopharmacologia* 4:247-260, 1963

Woodruff RA, Murphy GE and Herjanic M: The natural history of affective disorders. I. Symptoms of 72 patients at the time of index hospital admissions. *J Psychiatr Res* 5:255-263, 1967

2

Opiate Receptors and Opioid Peptides: Are They Involved in Drug Addiction?

ERIC J. SIMON

INTRODUCTION

The recent discoveries of the existence of opiate receptors and of endogenous opioid peptides in the central nervous system of animals and man have raised hopes that an understanding of the molecular mechanism of drug addiction may soon be achieved. It is clear from the title of this chapter that that day is not yet here. I will give a brief chronological review of the significant discoveries and developments and will then summarize recent research that bears on the possible involvement of the endogenous opioid system in drug addiction.

THE DISCOVERY OF OPIATE RECEPTORS

The hypothesis that narcotic analgesics must bind to highly specific sites or receptors in the central nervous system (CNS) in order to produce their many well-known responses has been held by some investigators for several decades. The evidence for the existence of such receptor sites was compelling. It consisted primarily of the remarkable stereospecificity and, for certain parts of the molecules, structural specificity displayed by many of the pharmacological actions of narcotic analgesic drugs.

As thousands of analogues of morphine were synthesized in search of the still mythical nonaddictive analgesic it became clear that one enantiomer of a racemic mixture (usually the levo-rotatory one) was generally much more active than the other. Moreover, some parts of the molecule could be drastically altered with relatively little change in potency, whereas tampering with certain regions had dramatic effects. The most interesting and best studied such region is the substituent on the tertiary nitrogen, one of the functional groups essential for narcotic analgesic activity.

When the methyl group is substituted by a larger alkyl group, eg, an allyl or cyclopropylmethyl group, analgesic potency is reduced and the drug takes on the new pharmacological role of a potent, specific antagonist against many of the actions of morphine and related narcotics. Some drugs have both agonist and antagonist properties, while others, such as naloxone and naltrexone (the N-allyl and N-cyclopropylmethyl analogues, resp. of oxymorphone), are "pure" antagonists. The synthesis of mixed agonist-antagonist drugs as candidates for analgesics with low addiction liability has been a major enterprise in pharmaceutical company laboratories in recent years. Moreover, the pure antagonist naltrexone, longer acting than naloxone, has shown some promise for the treatment of heroin addicts.

The kinds of specificities described above are most easily explained by interaction with binding sites that exhibit complementary specificity. The search for such specific binding sites or opiate receptors began in the 1950s and bore fruit in the early 1970s. It was easy to show binding of opiates to cell constituents (Van Praag, 1966) but to distinguish specific from nonspecific binding proved difficult.

It was the measurement of stereospecific binding that led to success. Ingoglia and Dole (1970) were the first to apply stereospecificity to the search for receptors by injecting l- and d-methadone into the lateral ventricle of rats, but found no difference in the rate of diffusion of the enantiomers. Goldstein et al (1971) devised a method for measuring stereospecific binding of ^{3}H-levorphanol in mouse brain homogenates. They reported that only 2 percent of the total binding was stereospecific and the properties and distribution of this binding turned out to be quite different from those of the subsequently discovered "receptors." Upon purification this binding material proved to be cerebroside sulfate.

In 1973 our laboratory (Simon et al, 1973) and those of Snyder (1973) and Terenius (1973), using modifications of the Goldstein procedure, independently and simultaneously, reported the observation in animal brain homogenates of stereospecific binding of opiates that represented the major portion of the total binding. Since that time stereospecific binding studies have been done in many laboratories and much evidence has been accumulated suggesting that these stereospecific sites are indeed receptors that are responsible for many of the pharmacological actions of the opiates. They have been found in man (Hiller et al, 1973) and in all vertebrates so far studied. Very recently it has been reported that they also exist in some invertebrates (Stefano, 1980).

PROPERTIES AND DISTRIBUTION OF OPIATE RECEPTORS

The properties of the opiate binding sites have been studied extensively and their distribution in the brain and spinal cord has been mapped in considerable detail by dissection and *in vitro* binding measurement (Hiller, 1973; Kuhar, 1973) as well as by autoradiography (Pert, 1975; Atweh, 1977; Atweh, 1977; Atweh, 1977).

Stereospecific binding is saturable and total binding amounts to 15–20 pmol of opiate per gram of rat brain. Affinities range from K_D of 0.25 nM for a potent fentanyl analogue (Stahl et al, 1977) to little or no affinity for drugs devoid of opiate activity. The average dissociation constants for effective narcotic analgesics are in the 1–10 nM range. The pH optimum for binding is in the physiological range with a fairly broad optimum between 6.5 and 8.0. The addition of salts to the incubation mixture tends to reduce binding. Sodium represents an interesting exception. Its presence causes inhibition of agonist binding, whereas the binding of most antagonists is significantly increased. This highly specific effect of sodium (exhibited to some extent by Li^+ but not by any of the other alkali metals, K^+, Rb^+, or Cs^+) has been shown in our laboratory to be the result of a conformational change in the opiate receptor (Simon et al, 1975).

The inhibition of stereospecific binding by proteolytic enzymes (Simon et al, 1973; Pasternak, 1973) and a variety of protein reagents, including sulfhydryl reagents, suggests the involvement of protein moieties in opiate binding. The role of phospholipids is yet to be established. Binding is inhibited by some, but not all, phospholipase A preparations (Simon et al, 1973; Pasternak, 1973) but not by phospholipases C or D. Moreover, we have shown (Lin, 1978) that inhibition by phospholipase A can be reversed by washing the membrane preparation with a solution of bovine serum albumin, suggesting that the nature of the phospholipid environment may be very important for the active conformation of the opiate receptor.

The extensive mapping studies can be summarized here only briefly. The highest levels of opiate receptors are found in the areas of the limbic system and in the regions that have been implicated in the pathways involved in pain perception and modulation, such as the periventricular and periaqueductal gray areas, the medial thalamus, the nucleus raphe magnus and the substantia gelatinosa of the spinal cord. It has been suggested that the limbic system receptors may be involved in opiate-induced euphoria (or dysphoria) and in the affective aspects of pain perception.

Perhaps the most convincing evidence suggesting that stereospecific binding has pharmacological relevance comes from a number of studies that show excellent correlation between pharmacological potencies and *in vitro* binding affinities for a large number of drugs, varying in analgesic potencies over 5-6 orders of magnitude (Stahl et al, 1977; Wilson et al, 1975).

DISCOVERY AND MAPPING OF ENDOGENOUS OPIOID PEPTIDES

The evidence that the brain of all vertebrates investigated, from the hagfish to man, contains opiate receptors led investigators to raise the question why such receptors for plant-derived substances exist in the CNS and have survived eons of evolution. A physiological role for opiate receptors that confers a selective advantage on the organisms seemed probable, suggesting the presence of an endogenous opiatelike ligand for the receptor. This notion was reinforced by the finding in the early 1970s that electrical stimulation of certain brain areas was able to mobilize an endogenous pain-relieving system, resulting in long-lasting analgesia (Reynolds, 1969; Mayer et al, 1971).

None of the many known neurotransmitters or neurohormones was found to exhibit high affinity for opiate receptors. A number of laboratories therefore initiated a search for new opiatelike substances in extracts of animal brain. This search was successful first in the laboratories of Hughes and Kosterlitz (1975) and of Terenius and Wahlström (1974). Goldstein and his collaborators (1975) at about the same time, reported opioid activity in extracts of pituitary glands. Hughes utilized the *in vitro* bioassays for opiates, namely naloxone-reversible inhibition of electrically evoked contraction of the mouse vas deferens or the guinea pig ileum, while Terenius assayed endogenous opioid activity by measuring ability of brain extracts and fractions to compete with labeled opiates for receptor binding.

These studies culminated in the identification of the opioid substances in extracts of pig brain by Hughes et al (1975). They reported that the activity resided in two pentapeptides, Tyr-Gly-Gly-Phe-Met and Tyr-Gly-Gly-Phe-Leu, which they named methionine (Met) and leucine (Leu) enkephalin. Hughes et al also reported the interesting observation that the sequence of Met-enkephalin was present as amino acid residues 61–65 in the pituitary hormone β-lipotropin (βLPH). This hormone had been isolated in 1965 from pituitary glands by C.H. Li (1964). It possessed weak lipolytic activity which was never seriously thought to be its real function. The report of Hughes et al, along with that of the Goldstein group of the existence of opioid activity in the pituitary gland, led Guillemin to examine the extracts of pig hypothalami and pituitary glands (remaining in his freezer from his Nobel prize winning identification of hypothalamic releasing factors). Two polypeptides with opioid activity were found and sequenced (Ling et al, 1976). They proved to have structures identical with amino acid sequences 61–76 and

61–77 of βLPH. Meanwhile, potent opioid activity was found in the C-terminal fragment of βLPH (LPH 61–91) in two laboratories (Bradbury et al, 1976; Cox et al, 1976) while the intact βLPH molecule was inactive. The proliferation of endogenous peptides with opioid activity caused the author of this paper to suggest the term "endorphin" (a contraction of "endogenous" and "morphine") which has been widely accepted. The C-terminal fragment was renamed β-endorphin by Li, while LPH 61–76 and 61–77 were named α and γ-endorphin, respectively, by Guillemin.

Recently, a number of additional peptides with opioid activity has been reported. One of the most important of these is a peptide from the pituitary characterized by A. Goldstein and collaborators (1979). The peptide was named dynorphin by the authors because of its potent opioid activity in bioassay systems. It has been found in certain areas of the CNS in addition to the pituitary.

All the opioid peptides exhibit opiatelike activity when injected intraventricularly. This activity includes analgesia, respiratory depression and a variety of behavioral changes including the production of a rigid catatonia. The pharmacological effects of the enkephalins are very fleeting, presumably due to their rapid destruction by peptidases. The longer-chain endorphins are more stable and produce long-lived effects. Thus, analgesia from intraventricular administration of β-endorphin can last 3–4 hours. All of the responses to endorphins are reversible by opiate antagonists, such as naloxone. There have been reports that certain analogues of enkephalin can produce analgesia after systemic injection or even oral ingestion (Roemer et al, 1977).

Distribution of enkephalins has been studied by biochemical (Simantov et al, 1976) as well as by bioassay (Hughes et al, 1977) and immunohistochemical techniques (Elde et al, 1976; Simantov et al, 1976). The distribution of enkephalins in the CNS shows considerable, though not complete, correlation with the distribution of opiate receptors. Thus, the globus pallidus has a very high density of enkephalin (or at least enkephalinlike immunoreactive material) while it is low in opiate receptors. Certain cortical areas dense in opiate receptors have low levels of enkephalin.

In the earlier studies of Hökfelt and colleagues (1976) the immunofluorescence was all found in nerve fibers and terminals but not in cell bodies. In a more recent paper, this group (Hökfelt et al, 1977) utilized colchicine which is known to arrest axonal transport. After such treatment it was possible to find immunofluorescence in cell bodies after treatment with antiserum to Met-enkephalin. More than 20 cell groups containing enkephalin have so far been observed in the brain and spinal cord, a number somewhat larger than the 15 catecholamine cell groups known to exist in rat brain. The authors felt that their results indicate that these perikarya possess the machinery for enkephalin biosynthesis. This was the first indication that enkephalin is probably not derived from large endorphin precursors, since levels of β-lipotropin and β-endorphin are very low in some of the areas that are found to have high enkephalin levels.

Studies on the distribution of β-endorphin in the laboratories of Guillemin (1977) and Watson (1977) have provided convincing evidence for a distribution that is very different from that of the enkephalins. This has led to the suggestion that the CNS has separate enkephalinergic and endorphiergic neuronal systems. β-endorphin is present in the pituitary, where there is little or no enkephalin, as well as in certain regions of the brain. Brain β-endorphin seems to originate in a single set of neurons located in the peri-arcuate region of the hypothalamus, with axons projecting throughout the brain stem and into areas of the forebrain.

NARCOTIC ADDICTION

There are a number of ways in which the endogenous opioid system might be involved in drug addiction. There could be changes in the number or properties of opiate receptors, altered levels of enkephalins and/or endorphins and finally changes in the metabolism of the opioid peptides. Experiments probing these possible changes will be summarized.

All opioid peptides will produce tolerance and physical dependence when injected repeatedly. Cross-tolerance with plant alkaloid opiates has also been shown. This does not prove that tolerance/dependence develop to endogenously produced and released endorphins nor that these peptides and their receptors are involved in the formation of tolerance and dependence to narcotics.

A theory that predated the biochemical demonstration of opiate receptors is one that suggests changes in either the number or binding characteristics of opiate receptors. A change in binding affinities similar to that seen when sodium concentration is increased during *in vitro* binding is especially attractive, since sensitivity to agonists decreases during tolerance formation while sensitivity to antagonists increases dramatically. Klee and Streaty (1974) examined this question in whole rat brain and found no changes in the number or affinities of opiate binding sites. We felt that this might be explicable by a "drowning out" of changes occurring in only a few brain regions. However, an examination of receptor number and binding affinities in the medial thalamus, periventricular gray region and caudate nucleus in collaboration with K. Bonnet (1976) gave equally negative results. Whereas these three areas have high levels of receptors and/or have been implicated in various aspects of opiate action, the possibility still remains that these were not the appropriate areas to examine. However, it is at least equally possible that detectable changes in receptors do not occur during chronic morphinization.

The absence of changes in opiate binding during chronic morphinization of animals has given rise to the notion that the alterations occur in steps subsequent to the binding of opiates to their receptor. Several years ago Collier and Roy (1974) reported that opiates inhibit prostaglandin E_1-stimulated adenylate cyclase in rat brain homogenate. This interesting observation has proved difficult to reproduce. However, a similar observation from studies in a cell culture system has lent credence and support to this finding. Neuroblastoma x glioma hybrid cells in culture were shown to contain opiate receptors (Sharma et al, 1975). The receptor binding of opiates and endogenous opioids results in inhibition of basal as well as prostaglandin E_1-stimulated adenylate cyclase. When these cultures are grown in the presence of morphine inhibition of adenylate cyclase requires increasing concentrations of opiates, a finding that has been suggested as the cellular equivalent of tolerance. It is due to an increase in enzyme activity that seems to be induced by the presence of opiate in the culture medium. Moreover, a putative cellular equivalent of withdrawal is also observed. When cells grown in morphine are placed in drug-free medium or treated with naloxone there is a dramatic overproduction of cyclic AMP (cAMP). The relevance of these results to the CNS of intact animals has yet to be established.

Observations of Collier and his collaborators provide further evidence that cAMP may play a role in chronic effects of opiates. Treatment of naive animals with inhibitors of phosphodiesterase, the enzyme that destroys cAMP, results in symptoms that closely resemble the withdrawal syndrome from opiates. This has been termed quasi morphine withdrawal syndrome (QMWS) by Collier who suggests that it results from increased brain levels of cAMP (1974).

The possibility that a change in endorphin level might be observed during tolerance/dependence development has also received attention. A report by Simantov and Snyder (1976) that enkephalin levels are elevated in brains of tolerant rats has been refuted by experiments from the same laboratory (1977). The earlier work which had been done using a radioreceptor assay was not supported when the much more specific radioimmunoassay was used.

Herz's group (1979) found little change in the level of β-endorphin immunoreactivity 10 days after morphine pellet implantation in rats. However, when the period of exposure to morphine was extended to one month or longer a 60 percent decrease of β-endorphin-like immunoreactivity from the intermediate/posterior lobe of the pituitary was observed. There was also a decrease in some brain areas such as septum and midbrain, but the level in the hypothalamus was unaltered. Some decrease in enkephalin levels in the striatum and the pituitary was also reported. The authors admit that interpretation of these data is difficult, especially since attempts to repeat these experiments with the potent narcotic analgesic etorphine were unsuccessful and since the period of pellet implantation far exceeded the period required for the development of tolerance and physical dependence.

Recently there has been a report (Su et al, 1978) that the intravenous administration of 4 mg of human β-endorphin to human addicts led to dramatic improvement in severe abstinence syndromes. There was no euphoria and little adverse effect. In a double-blind study it was found that subjects were able to distinguish morphine and β-endorphin. After endorphin treatment they felt thirsty, dizzy, sleepy, warm, and had "a strange feeling throughout the body." However, all these symptoms disappeared in 20 minutes whereas the beneficial effects of endorphin on the withdrawal syndrome lasted for several days. The long-lasting suppression of especially the most severe symptoms of abstinence (vomiting, diarrhea, tremor, and restlessness) by a single dose of β-endorphin suggested to the authors the possibility that this endogenous peptide may indeed have a role in the mechanism of tolerance/dependence development to opiates.

An exciting recent discovery that could have a bearing on our understanding of the role of the endogenous opioid system in addiction was made simultaneously in Paris and at Stanford University. Malfroy et al (1978) and Sullivan et al (1978) reported the existence of a membrane-bound peptidase that appears to be relatively specific for the breakdown of enkephalins. This "enkephalinase" is a carboxydipeptidase, ie, it splits enkephalin between the glycine in position 3 and the phenylalanine. The Schwartz group reported that the level of this enzyme increases significantly during chronic morphinization of rats. Other groups have found less dramatic changes, but this finding deserves watching. An enzyme, called by the authors enkephalinase A, has recently been purified by Gorenstein et al (1980).

A recent study of plasma β-endorphin levels in narcotic addicts and non-addict control subjects showed a large decrease of plasma β-endorphin in the addicts (Ho et al, 1980). However, the antiserum used for the radioimmunoassays must have been rather non-specific, since the control levels of β-endorphin were about 1000 pg/ml plasma. Many other laboratories have reported anywhere from borderline detectable levels to 30 pg/ml.

For completeness I should like to mention two recent developments of considerable interest for which the relationship to the opiate receptor is still unknown.

Walter et al (1978) reported that it was possible to suppress the abstinence syndrome when rats were withdrawn from chronic morphine by administration of the dipeptide Z-Pro-D-Leu. There was no effect on the analgesic response to morphine. The mechanism of this phenomenon is not understood.

Based on the abundant literature which seems to implicate catecholamines in the actions of opiates, Gold et al (1978) treated human heroin addicts with clonidine. In a double-blind, placebo-controlled study clonidine eliminated objective signs and subjective symptoms of opiate withdrawal for 4–6 hours in all addicts. In an open pilot study the same patients did well while taking clonidine for one week. All of the patients had been addicted to opiates for 6–10 years and had been on methadone for 6–60 months at the time of the study. The authors suggest that their success with clonidine indicates that abstinence may be produced by an interaction between opiate receptors and alpha-2 adrenergic receptors in the mediation of effects by endogenous opiates in noradrenergic areas such as the locus coeruleus.

CONCLUDING COMMENTS

In spite of the enormous activity in research on opiate receptors and endorphins, the physiological function of this system has not yet been established. Involvement of the endogenous opioid system has been suggested for pain suppression, narcotic addiction, mental diseases, in particular, schizophrenia and depression, sexual activity, and overeating. Proof is not yet available for any of these roles. The best evidence exists for an involvement of endogenous opioids and their receptors in the modulation of pain. It is based primarily on the observation that several types of nondrug induced analgesias, such as electrical stimulation analgesia, acupuncture and placebo analgesia are reversible by naloxone. The release of enkephalins and β-endorphin into CSF during analgesia has also been reported.

As can be seen from the above summary, evidence for the participation of the endogenous opioid system in narcotic addiction is still very sparse and largely indirect. Moreover, the changes that have been reported deal with a possible involvement in the development of tolerance and physical dependence Evidence for a role of the endorphin system in such important aspects of drug abuse as psychic dependence and drug hunger is even more difficult to obtain.

Nevertheless, there is considerable optimism among researchers in this field. This optimistic outlook is based in part on the conviction that it is highly improbable that endogenous opioid peptides would not be involved in the actions of exogenous opiates, which they resemble so closely in their pharmacology. If opiate receptors are involved in the acute effects of opiates (for which the evidence is much better) then why should they not have a role in the chronic effects of the same drugs?

Moreover, the evidence cited, while admittedly unconvincing, is sufficiently "teasing" to encourage further research along these lines. One of the reasons for the slow progress in this area to date is the lack of appropriate research tools, many of which are just now becoming available. Thus, we are just beginning to understand the biosynthesis and metabolic fate of opioid peptides. This knowledge is essential to a recognition of alterations in the metabolism or turnover of the peptides during chronic morphinization.

When it was found that there are no changes in opiate receptors there was no awareness that several different subclasses of opiate receptors exist (see chapter by Dr. R.S. Zukin for a discussion of multiple opiate receptors). A similar statement applies to the measurement of opioid peptides. Only the enkephalins and β-endorphin have been measured, yet several other peptides have since been found to exist.

Thus, I wish to terminate this discussion on an upbeat note by making the prediction that an involvement of the opiate receptor–opioid peptide system in the biochemical mechanism of opiate addiction will be delineated within the next few years. It is not beyond the realm of possibility that a role for this system may also be found in certain other types of substance abuse or compulsive behavior.

REFERENCES

Atweh SF and Kuhar MF: Autoradiographic localization of opiate receptors in rat brain. I. Spinal cord and lower medulla. *Brain Res* 124:53–67, 1977

Atweh SF and Kuhar MJ: Autoradiographic localization of opiate receptors in rat brain. II. The brainstem. *Brain Res* 129:1–12, 1977

Atweh SF and Kuhar MJ: Autoradiographic localization of opiate receptors in rat brain. III. The telencephalon. *Brain Res* 134:393–406, 1977

Bonnet KA, Hiller JM and Simon EJ: The effects of chronic opiate treatment and social isolation on opiate receptors in rodent brain. In: *Opiates and Endogenous Opioid Peptides*. Proceedings of the International Narcotic Research Conference Meeting, Aberdeen, UK. Amsterdam, North Holland, 1976 p 335–343

Bradbury AF, Smyth DG, Snell CR, Birdsall NJM and Hulme EC: C fragment of lipotropin has a high affinity for brain opiate receptors. *Nature* 260:793–799, 1976

Childers SR, Simantov R and Snyder SH: Enkephalin: Radioimmunoassay and radio-receptor assay in morphine dependent rats. *Eur J Pharmacol* 46:289–293, 1977

Collier HOJ, Francis DL, Henderson G and Schneider S: Quasi morphine abstinence syndrome. *Nature* 249:471–473, 1974

Collier HOJ and Roy AC: Morphine-like drugs inhibit the stimulation by E prostaglandins of cyclic AMP formation by rat brain homogenate. *Nature* 248:24–27, 1974

Cox BM, Goldstein A and Li CH: Opioid activity of a peptide β-lipotropin-(61–91), derived from β-lipotropin. *Proc Natl Acad Sci USA* 73:1821–1823, 1976

Elde R, Hökfelt T, Johansson O and Terenius L: Immunohistochemical studies using antibodies to leucine-enkephalin: Initial observations on the nervous system of the rat. *Neuroscience* 1:349–351, 1976

Gold M, Redmond DE Jr and Kleber HD: Clonidine blocks acute opiate-withdrawal symptoms. *Lancet* 16:599–601, 1978

Goldstein A, Lowney LI and Pal BK: Stereospecific and nonspecific interactions of the morphine congener levorphanol in subcellular fractions of mouse brain. *Proc Nat Acad Sci USA* 68:1742-1747, 1971

Goldstein A, Tachibana S, Lowney LI, Hunkapiller M and Hood L: Dynorphin (1-13), an extraordinarily potent opioid peptide. *Proc Natl Acad Sci USA* 76:6666-6670, 1979

Gorenstein C and Snyder SH: Characterization of enkephalinases. In: Way EL (ed.) *Endogenous and Exogenous Opiate Agonists and Antagonists.* New York, Pergamon, 1980 p 345-348

Herz A, Höllt V and Przewlocki R: Endogenous opioids and addiction. In: Wuttke W, Weindl A, Voigt KH and Fries RR (eds.) *Brain and Pituitary Peptides.* Basel, S Karger, 1979 p 183-189

Hiller JM, Pearson J and Simon EJ: Distribution of stereospecific binding of the potent narcotic analgesic etorphine in the human brain: predominance in the limbic system. *Res Commun Chem Pathol Pharmacol* 6:1052-1062, 1973

Ho WKK, Wen HL and Ling N: Beta-endorphin-like immunoreactivity in the plasma of heroin addicts and normal subjects. *Neuropharmacology* 19:117-120, 1980

Hökfelt T, Elde R, Johansson O, Terenius L and Stein L: The distribution of enkephalin-immunoreactive cell bodies in the rat central nervous system. *Neurosci Lett* 5:25-31, 1977

Hughes J: Isolation of an endogenous compound from the brain with properties similar to morphine. *Brain Res* 88:295-308, 1975

Hughes J, Kosterlitz HW and Smith TW: The distribution of methionine-enkephalin and leucine-enkephalin in the brain and peripheral tissues. *Brit J Pharmacol* 61:639-647, 1977

Hughes J, Smith TW, Kosterlitz H, Fothergill LA, Morgan BA and Morris HR: Identification of two related pentapeptides from the brain with potent opiate agonist activity. *Nature* 258:577-579, 1975

Ingoglia NA and Dole VP: Localization of d and l-methadone after intraventricular injection into rat brains. *J Pharmacol Exp Therap* 175:84-87, 1970

Klee WA and Streaty RA: Narcotic receptor sites in morphine-dependent rats. *Nature* 248:61-63. 1974

Kuhar MJ, Pert CB and Snyder SH: Regional distribution of opiate receptor binding in monkey and human brain. *Nature* 245:447-450, 1973

Li CH: Lipotropin: A new active peptide from pituitary glands. *Nature* 201:924, 1964

Lin H-K and Simon EJ: Phospholipase A inhibition of opiate receptor binding can be reversed by albumin. *Nature* 271:383-384, 1978

Ling J, Burgus R and Guillemin R: Isolation, primary structure, and synthesis of α-endorphin and γ-endorphin, two peptides of hypothalamic-hypophysial origin with morphinomimetic activities. *Proc Natl Acad Sci USA* 73:3942-3946, 1976

Malfroy B, Swerts JP, Guyon A, Roques BP and Schwartz JC: High-affinity enkephalin-degrading peptidase in brain is increased after morphine. *Nature* 26:523-526, 1978

Mayer DJ, Wolfle TL, Akil H, Carder B and Liebeskind JC: Analgesia from electrical stimulation in the brain stem of the rat. *Science* 174:1351-1354, 1971

Pasternak GW and Snyder SH: Opiate receptor binding: Effects of enzymatic treatment. *Mol Pharmacol* 10:183-193, 1973

Pert CB, Kuhar MJ and Snyder SH: Autoradiographic localization of the opiate receptor in rat brain. *Life Sci* 16:1849-1854, 1975

Pert CB and Snyder SH: Opiate receptor: demonstration in nervous tissue. *Science* 179:1011-1014, 1973

Reynolds DV: Surgery in the rat during electrical analgesia induced by focal brain stimulation. *Science* 164:444–445, 1969

Roemer D, Buescher HH, Hill RC, Pless J, Bauer W, Cardinaux F, Closse A, Hauser D and Huguenin R: A synthetic enkephalin analogue with prolonged parenteral and oral analgesic activity. *Nature* 268:547–549, 1977

Rossier J, Vargo TM, Minick S, Long N, Bloom FE and Guillemin R: Regional dissociation of beta-endorphin and enkephalin contents in rat brain and pituitary. *Proc Natl Acad Sci USA* 74:5162–5165, 1977

Sharma SK, Nirenberg M and Klee WA: Morphine receptors as regulators of adenylate cyclase activity. *Proc Natl Acad Sci USA* 72:590–594, 1975

Simantov R, Kuhar MJ, Pasternak GW and Snyder SH: The regional distribution of a morphine-like factor enkephalin in monkey brain. *Brain Res* 106:189–197, 1976

Simantov R, Kuhar MJ, Uhl GR and Snyder SH: Opioid peptide enkephalin: Immunohistochemical mapping in rat central nervous system. *Proc Natl Acad Sci USA* 74:2167–2171, 1977

Simantov R and Snyder SH: Elevated levels of enkephalin in morphine-dependent rats. *Nature* 262:505–507, 1976

Simon EJ, Hiller JM and Edelman I: Stereospecific binding of the potent narcotic analgesic ^{3}H-etorphine to rat brain homogenate. *Proc Nat Acad Sci USA* 70:1947–1949, 1973

Simon EJ and Groth J: Kinetics of opiate receptor inactivation by sulfhydryl reagents: Evidence for conformational change in presence of sodium ions. *Proc Natl Acad Sci USA* 72:2404–2407, 1975

Stahl KD, van Bever W, Janssen P and Simon EJ: Receptor affinity and pharmacological potency of a series of narcotic analgesic, antidiarrheal and neuroleptic drugs. *Eur J Pharmacol* 46:199–205, 1977

Stefano GB, Kream RM and Zukin RS: Demonstration of stereospecific opiate binding in the nervous tissue of the marine mollusc Mytilis edulis. *Brain Res* 181:440–445, 1980

Su CY, Lin SH, Wang YT, Li CH, Hung LH, Lin CS and Lin BC: Effects of β-endorphin on narcotic abstinence syndrome in man. *J Formos Med Assoc* 77:133–141, 1978

Sullivan S, Akil H and Barchas JD: In vitro degradation of enkephalin: Evidence for cleavage at the Gly-Phe bond. *Commun Psychopharmacol* 2:525–531, 1978

Terenius L: Stereospecific interaction between narcotic analgesics and a synaptic plasma membrane fraction of rat cerebral cortex. *Acta Pharmacol Toxicol* 32:317–320, 1973

Terenius L and Wahlström A: Inhibitor(s) of narcotic receptor binding in brain extracts and cerebrospinal fluid. *Acta Pharmacol Toxicol* 35:Suppl 1 55, 1974

Teschemacher H, Opheim KE, Cox BM and Goldstein A: A peptide-like substance from pituitary that acts like morphine. I. Isolation. *Life Sci* 16:1771–1776, 1975

Van Praag D and Simon EJ: Studies on the intracellular distribution and tissue binding of dihydromorphine-7,8-^{3}H in the rat. *Proc Soc Exp Biol Med* 122:6–11, 1966

Walter R, Ritzmann RF, Bhargava HN, Rainbow TC, Flexner LB and Krivoy WA: Inhibition by Z-Pro-D-Leu of development of tolerance to and physical dependence on morphine in mice. *Proc Natl Acad Sci USA* 75:4573–4576, 1978

Watson SJ, Barchas JD and Li CH: β-lipotropin: Localization of cells and axons in rat brain by immunocytochemistry. *Proc Natl Acad Sci USA* 74:5155–5158, 1977

Wilson RS, Rogers MF, Pert CB and Snyder SH: Homologous N-alkylnorketobemidones. Correlation of receptor binding with analgesic potency. *J Med Chem* 18:240–242, 1975

3

Applications of Human Behavioral Pharmacology to the Problems of Drug Addicts: A Brief Review

CHARLES P. O'BRIEN
JOSEPH W. TERNES
ROBERT GREENSTEIN
GEORGE E. WOODY

The work of Abraham Wikler (1973) over the past three decades has called attention to the importance of conditioned responses in the addictive process. Drugs act as powerful forces in shaping behavior, both by their direct pleasant effects (positive reinforcement) and by their effects in relieving withdrawal symptoms (negative reinforcement). Wikler theorized that the environmental cues which have been repeatedly paired with drug-induced states may become conditioned stimuli. He observed that former addicts who are free of drugs often develop tearing and yawning (opiate withdrawal signs) when they discuss drugs in group therapy. He and others subsequently showed that withdrawal signs could become conditioned in animals (Wikler and Pescor, 1967; Goldberg and Schuster, 1970). More recently, conditioned withdrawal has been demonstrated in humans (O'Brien et al, 1975; O'Brien et al, 1977). These conditioned withdrawal responses are thought to be partly due to simple pairing of pharmacological withdrawal with environmental cues, and partly due to pairing of environmental stimuli with the body's homeostatic mechanisms adapting to the onset of drug effects (Wikler, 1973; Siegel, 1974). Eventually the environmental stimuli themselves can elicit the adaptative response and this can be perceived as withdrawal.

As a result of this conditioning former addicts may develop withdrawal symptoms when they return to the environment in which they had previously used drugs. Not only do they develop drug-craving, but actual physical signs of sickness may occur (tearing, yawning, nausea, vomiting). There is also some evidence (Whitehead, 1974; O'Brien, 1975) that conditioned withdrawal can occur in patients maintained on a steady dose of methadone.

There are other conditioning factors which help to maintain self-administration of drugs. Addicts tend to use drugs in a ritualistic fashion. When the drug is administered, the withdrawal discomfort (both pharmacological and conditioned) is eased. At times, depending on the level of tolerance and dose of the drug used, the patient will feel euphoric. There is some controversy over how often a typical addict obtains euphoria rather than just relief of withdrawal distress (McAulliffee and Gordon, 1974), but clearly the reward is intermittant. Since intermittant reinforcement is very effective in maintaining behavior, this may explain why self-administration can continue when street heroin potency is low or when saline is substituted for opiate (O'Brien, 1975). Addicts who report pleasure from self-injection of inactive substances have been termed "needle freaks" (Levine, 1974). This phenomenon is usually seen only in "blind" conditions when the user expects a drug effect, but the substance administered actually contains little or no active drug. If addicts are informed that a substance is a placebo or if they know they are on an antagonist which will block drug effects, self-injection will stop after a few trials (Altman et al, 1976).

The existence of these conditioned phenomena requires that they be considered in the treatment of addiction. A number of innovative methods have been attempted which might influence conditioning or enable the patient to cope with conditioned withdrawal or conditioned drug craving.

COUNTERCONDITIONING PROCEDURES

Numerous published studies have described procedures to combat drug-taking behavior by aversive conditioning. These have been critically reviewed by Callner (1975). The reports consist of single cases or groups of cases, some with excellent results. Electrical and chemical aversion techniques are difficult to apply to typical addicts, and the method of covert conditioning (Cautela, 1975) has gained some acceptance.

Covert conditioning or sensitization consists of the use of imagined scenes as aversive events and as rewarding events. Beginning with the initial craving for drugs the patient is asked to imagine as clearly as possible each link in the chain of events leading to drug-taking. Instead of pleasant drug effects, the patient is asked to imagine becoming severely ill in vivid terms as a consequence of the drug. When the patient imagines the avoidance of drugs he is told to imagine pleasant scenes. Covert sensitization has been successfully used in several published case reports or series of cases (Wisocki, 1973; Cautela and Rosenstein, 1975). It has been used in combination with other behavioral techniques (O'Brien et al, 1972) and it has been successfully augmented by hypnosis (Copeman, 1977) and by chemical aversion (Maletzky, 1974).

EXTINCTION OR DESENSITIZATION PROCEDURES

One approach to treatment is to attempt the systematic extinction of conditioned responses which have developed throughout the course of addiction. This method directly follows from the assumption that conditioned responses are helping to maintain drug-taking behavior. Thus an attempt to extinguish these responses would appear logical. To accomplish this, exposure to the situations associated with drug-taking should be accomplished, but drug effects must not follow. Kraft (1970) in a series of case reports of amphetamine-barbiturate users found certain social situations to provoke drug-taking. His treatment consisted of setting up hierarchies of such situations for each patient (Wolpe, 1958) and exposing the patient to each one beginning with the least evocative situation. Hypnosis and relaxation were used to prevent the patient from responding in the usual way with anxiety and drug-ingestion. Although definition of population and follow-up were minimal (Kraft, 1976), the results were encouraging.

Our group (O'Brien, 1975) has been able to obtain (by behavioral interview) hierarchies of stimuli which provoke craving or withdrawal responses among addicts. When slides or video tapes of these situations were shown to addict patients, the response was variable. Some reported strong drug-craving and others reported no effects (O'Brien et al, 1974). In subsequent studies we have thus far failed to find stimuli which are consistently effective. Negative affectual responses and slight feelings of withdrawal have been reported by Teasdale (1973) when drug related slides were shown to addicts. Physiological changes in response to video tapes of drug taking behavior have been reported by Sideroff and Jarvik (1977).

We have conducted several studies of detoxified opiate addicts and control subjects under baseline conditions in a controlled environment. While some addicts showed conditioned withdrawal responses to slides and video tapes of drug-related activities, more consistent responses occurred when the subjects handled bags of heroin or went through pre-injection rituals ("cook-up"). Conditioned withdrawal responses were: decreases in skin temperature, increases in heart rate, increases in pupil size, and increased scores on withdrawal and craving ratings (O'Brien et al, Note 1). If a simple technique could be found for producing conditioned craving or withdrawal in the clinic, patients could be systematically desensitized. Of course, it is not certain how much generalization there would be to the natural environment. For optimum effectiveness, it might be necessary for patients to be desensitized in situations that clearly resemble their own neighborhoods.

Narcotic antagonists have also been considered as an aid to extinction of drug conditioned responses (Wikler, 1974). While a patient is receiving an antagonist, such as naltrexone, he is effectively "protected" from most of the effects of injected opiates. Thus he can be exposed to stimuli which provoke opiate use and even use opiates with little or no reinforcement. However, most patients who are maintained on narcotic antagonists rarely test them by injecting heroin. This is confirmed by urine tests as well as by patients reports (Kleber et al, 1974; O'Brien et al, 1974). The patients report that once they are convinced that opiate effects will be blocked by the antagonist, they do not wish to waste their money by using heroin. Since the addicts do not perform the rituals which usually precede drug-taking, they do not actually extinguish the conditioned responses associated with this behavior.

Another problem is that duration of treatment with naltrexone is usually fairly brief (National Research Council, 1978) and thus opportunities for extinction are limited. The antagonist is lacking in the reinforcing properties found in agonist such as methadone. It produces no euphoria and no physical dependence. In the absence of pharmacological reinforcement, small monetary rewards have been recommended to induce patients to continue ingesting naltrexone (Meyer et al, 1976). We have found the scheduling of the monetary reward to be important (Grabowski et al, 1978, Note 2). Both response-based schedules (continuous reinforcement, fixed ratio, variable ratio) and a time-based schedule (fixed interval) were compared. The contingency payments (a total of $40 per month for all schedules) produced a significant lengthening of duration of naltrexone treatment. The fixed ratio condition ($3.34 every third visit) was found to be optimal. Although the contingency payments produced a clear effect on treatment duration, our preliminary follow-up data suggest that active extinction of conditioned responses is necessary to improve overall treatment success rate.

How can former addicts be induced to go through pre-injection rituals while protected by naltrexone? Meyer et al (1976) have reported that hospitalized former addicts on naltrexone usually did not continue to inject heroin spontaneously even when the drug is readily available at minimal cost. They did resume injecting when naltrexone was stopped. Our group (O'Brien et al, 1974; O'Brien, 1975) has attempted to actively extinguish pre-injection rituals and self-injection behavior as an experimental treatment. Former addicts maintained on antagonist (cyclazocine or naltrexone) were given opiates to self-inject on a regular prescribed basis in the laboratory. The behavior of these addicts changed remarkably over 5 to 25 self-injections and this occurred whether the injections contained saline or opiate (double-blind). The entire procedure (including pre- and post-injection rituals) was reported as mildly pleasant after the first several injections. The pre-injection rituals themselves produced craving and withdrawal as measured by rating scales and physiological responses. The injection itself relieved withdrawal and produced weak opioid effects on the first several occasions. As extinction progressed, the withdrawal responses increased and were worsened rather than relieved by the self-injection. Some patients became angry and many refused to continue the injections despite cash inducements.

Although the blocked self-injections resulted in the patients' no longer enjoying the drug-taking rituals, it was found that long-term outcome did not appear to have been affected. Recently, however, we have analyzed data from 118 patients who were followed-up at one month and six months after stopping naltrexone (O'Brien et al, Note 3). Ninety-seven patients received naltrexone and no behavioral treatment. Twenty-one were randomly assigned to self-injection ("extinction") using either an opiate (hydromorphone) or saline under double-blind conditions. There were no significant differences among treatment groups in age, education, sex, duration of addiction, criminal involvement, or prior treatment history. All patients received supportive counseling during treatment. The duration of treatment was approximately 60 days for all treatment groups except for those who self-injected saline. The saline group more rapidly developed craving and with-drawal responses and dropped out of treatment after a mean of only 31 days. Six months after stopping treatment, approximately 84 percent of patients were located for a follow-up interview, and urine test. Outcome was determined by employment, drug use, criminal activity, and social functioning measures. Patients who self-injected opiate in the laboratory while "blocked" by naltrexone had a significantly better outcome than controls who received no behavior therapy. Those who received saline had a significantly worse outcome than controls.

These results are only preliminary; they must be replicated by a larger study which eliminates some of the flaws in the initial study. The data suggest, however, that attempts to extinguish putative conditioned responses in opiate addicts can have beneficial effects or detrimental effects depending on how extinction procedures are applied. We are now testing a more gradual desensitization procedure which may lead to longer treatment duration and better outcome.

CONCLUSION

There is considerable evidence from animal and human studies that conditioning plays a role in maintaining drug-seeking behavior. Systematic efforts to modify drug conditioned bheavior as a therapeutic modality are still in their early stages. Although the initial results are promising, it must be remembered that human drug addiction is a complex process involving political and social as well as psychological and pharmacological factors. Behavioral treatments must be accompanied by broad rehabilitative measures.

NOTES

1. O'Brien CP, Ternes J and Greenstein R: Conditioned responses to drug-related stimuli in addicts and former addicts. (Manuscript in preparation)
2. Grabowski J, O'Brien CP, Greenstein R, Long M, Steinberg-Donato, S and Ternes J: Effects of contingent payment on compliance with a naltrexone regiman. (Manuscript in preparation)
3. O'Brien CP, Greenstein R, McLellan T, Ternes J and Woody G: Follow-up of opiate addicts treated by naltrexone and extinction of conditioned responses. (Manuscript in preparation)

REFERENCES

Altman JL, Meyer RE, Mirin SM and McNamee HB: Opiate antagonists and the modification of heroin self-administration behavior in man. *Int J Addiction* 11(3):485–499, 1976

Callner DA: Behavioral treatment approaches to drug abuse: A critical review of the research. *Psychol Bull* 82:143–164, 1975

Cautela JR and Rosenstein AK: The use of covert conditioning in the treatment of drug abuse. *Int J Addiction* 10:277–303, 1975

Copemann CD: Treatment of polydrug abuse and addiction by covert sensitization: Some contraindications. *Int J Addictions* 12:17–23, 1977

Goldberg SR and Schuster CR: Conditioned nalorphine-induced abstinence changes; persistence in post-morphine dependent monkeys. *J Exper Anal Behav* 14:33–46, 1970

Kleber H, Kinsella JK, Riordan C, Greaves S and Sweney D: The use of cyclozocine in treating narcotic addicts in a low-intervention setting. *Arch Gen Psychiatry* 30:37–42, 1974

Kraft T: Treatment of drinamyl addiction. *J Nerv Ment Disorder* 150:138–144, 1970

Kraft T: Long-term effects of behavior therapy. *Br J Psychiatry* 510–511, 1976

Lal H, Miksic S and Smith N: Naloxone antagonism of conditioned hyperthermia: An evidence for release of endogenous opioid. *Life Science* 18:971–976, 1976

Levine, DG: Needle freaks: Compulsive self-injection by drug users. *Am J Psychiatry* 131:297–299, 1974

Maletzky BM: Assisted covert sensitization for drug abuse. *Int J Addictions* 9:411–429, 1974

McAulliffee WE and Gordon RA: A test of Lindesmith's theory of addiction: The frequency of euphoria among long-term addicts. *Am J Sociol* 79:795–840, 1974

Meyer R, Randall M, Barrington C, Mirin S and Greenberg I: Limitations of an extinction approach to narcotic antagonist treatment. *Nat Inst Drug Abuse, Res Mon Series* (9):123–135, 1976

National Research Committee: Clinical evaluation of naltrexone treatment of opiate dependent individuals. *Arch Gen Psychiatry* 35:355–340, 1978

O'Brien CP: Experimental analysis of conditioning factors in human narcotic addiction. *Pharmacl Rev* 27:533–543, 1975

O'Brien CP, Chaddock B, Woody G and Greenstein R: Systematic extinction of narcotic drug use using narcotic antagonists. *Pro NAS/NRC Com Probl Drug Depend* 216–222, Washington, D.C., 1974

O'Brien CP, O'Brien TJ, Mintz J and Brady JP: Conditioning of narcotic abstinence symptoms in human subjects. *Drug Alco Depend* 115-123, 1975

O'Brien CP, Testa T, O'Brien TJ, Brady JP and Wells B: Narcotic withdrawal in humans. *Science* 195:1000-1002, 1977

O'Brien JS, Raynes AE and Patch VD: Treatment of heroin addiction with aversion therapy relaxation training and systematic desitization. *Behav Res Ther* 10:77-80, 1972

Sideroff SI and Jarvik ME: Conditioned responses to a video tape showing heroin related stimuli. *Pro Nat Drug Con Drug Abuse* May 5-9, 1977, (in press)

Siegal S: Evidence from rats that morphine tolerance is a learned response. *J Compar Physiol Psych* 89(5):498-506, 1975

Teasdale JD: Conditioned abstinence in narcotic addicts. *Int J Addictions* 8:274-292, 1974

Whitehead C: Methadone pseudowithdrawal syndrome: Paradign for a psycho-pharmacological model of opiate addiction. *Psychosom Med* 35:189-198, 1974

Wikler A: Dynamics of drug dependence. *Arch General Psychiatry* 28:611-616, 1973

Wikler A: Conditioning of successive adaptive responses to the initial effects of drugs. *Conditional Reflex* 8:193-210, 1973

Wikler A: Requirements for extinction of relapse—facilitating variables and for rehabilitation in a narcotic antagonist treatment program. In: *Narcotic Antagonists*, MC Braude, et al (eds), New York: Raven Press, 339-414, 1974

Wikler A and Prescor F: Classical conditioning of a morphine abstinence phenomenon, reinforcement of opioid-drinking behavior and "relapse" in morphine-addicted rats. *Psychopharmacologia* 10:255-284, 1967

Wisocki PA: The successful treatment of a heroin addict by covert conditioning techniques. *J Behav Ther Experi Psychiatry* 4:55-61, 1973

Wolpe J: *Psychotherapy by Reciprocal Inhibition*, pp 139-165. Stanford, California: Stanford University Press, 1958

4

Conditioned Taste Aversions and the Regulation of Drug-Taking Behavior

IAN P. STOLERMAN

INTRODUCTION

Considerable progress in the understanding of behavioral factors in drug dependence was made after methods were described for inducing animals to administer drugs to themselves. This development led to a new emphasis on the direct study of drug-taking behavior under controlled conditions, and it very effectively complemented the information obtained with the traditional pharmacological and psychiatric approaches, as well as challenging some common assumptions.

Researchers studying drug self-administration in animals have frequently interpreted their findings within an operant conditioning framework where the behavior is said to be maintained by positive reinforcing effects of the drugs. Many people have found it difficult to accept that some of the same self-administered drugs are extremely effective agents for producing the phenomenon called conditioned taste aversion (CTA). Drugs such as amphetamine, morphine, and chlordiazepoxide, which are known to serve reinforcing stimulus functions in self-administration experiments are also able to serve as the unconditioned, presumably aversive, stimulus in CTA studies. These super-ficially "paradoxical" effects need not be considered surprising in view of other evidence that the same nondrug stimulus can serve either reinforcing or aversive functions according to the circumstances (Morse and Kelleher, 1977), and in view of the multiple actions exerted by nearly all drugs.

This article reviews some research into CTA which was aimed at clarifying its relevance to drug dependence and to our understanding of how drugs could apparently serve multiple stimulus functions depending on the circumstances surrounding their administration. Although the problem is still unresolved, the work carried out to date exemplifies an analytical approach which has been used in many areas of behavioral pharmacology where drugs have varying and complex effects depending on behavioral and pharmacological variables. The work to be considered has suggested new directions for studies both of self-administration and of CTA, and has also challenged the usual interpretation of CTA in terms of drug-produced illness or toxicity. Identifying the specific variables involved when the same drug can either maintain or suppress responding may eventually make a substantial contribution to knowledge of the conditions under which dependence is most likely to develop. The possible implications of CTA for self-administration research will therefore be discussed. Stoleman and D'Mello (1981) have provided a more detailed account of this work.

CONDITIONED TASTE AVERSIONS PRODUCED BY NALOXONE

While many behavioral pharmacologists were busily applying the ideas and techniques of operant conditioning to the analysis of drug dependence, a different group of workers was engaged in the intensive study of CTA. In these latter experiments, changes in the consumption of distinctive foods or liquids were taken as evidence for the aversive properties of noxious events such as radiation sickness or emetic drugs (most often lithium or apomorphine salts). Provocative reviews describing much of the earlier work on CTA were written by Garcia and Ervin (1968) and by Revusky and Garcia (1970).

An example of CTA techniques in the behavioral analysis of morphine dependence can be found in the work of Pilcher and Stolerman (1976 a,b). Both the natural and the antagonist-precipitated morphine abstinence syndromes had been much studied, at least in part because prevention or termination of abstinent states may be involved in the reinforcement of self-administration behavior. The experiments summarized here were carried out to examine the possible value of CTA as a technique for assessing any aversive property of precipitated abstinence in rats repeatedly treated with morphine. The clear evidence that the narcotic antagonist naloxone could actually control behavior by acting as an aversive event in morphine-dependent rhesus monkeys was a major stimulus for this work (Goldberg et al, 1971).

Rats were allowed access to fluid for 1 hour only each day (normally 13.00–14.00 hr). After a period of adaptation to this regimen, one of two distinctively-flavored solutions was presented for 1hr on test days. Immediately after the flavored solutions were removed, the rats were injected intraperitoneally with either naloxone or saline solutions (flavor-injection "pairing"). For half of the rats, one flavor was repeatedly paired with naloxone, whereas the other flavor was repeatedly paired with saline. The flavor-injection pairings were reversed in the remaining rats, thus ensuring that effects due to the unconditioned palatabilities of the flavors were balanced out in the averaged results.

In rats maintained chronically on morphine (5 mg/kg ip) given twice daily at 09.30 and 17.30 hours, naloxone (10 mg/kg) induced very strong CTA. There were no substantial differences between the initial intakes of the naloxone- and the saline-paired flavors. On trial 2, there was a decrease in the intake of those flavors which had been paired with naloxone (10 mg/kg) on trial 1, as compared with the intake of saline-paired flavors by the same rats. Further, very marked decreases in intake were seen in subsequent trials.

It was also possible to induce clear CTA in rats chronically treated with nalorphine, a narcotic partial agonist, whereas much weaker CTA was induced with naloxone in rats which had received neither morphine nor nalophine. The greatly enhanced effectiveness of naloxone in the rats chronically treated with morphine or nalorphine suggested that precipitated abstinence reactions were the major events inducing the CTA in these rats. It seemed, therefore, that the CTA technique provided a means for assessing the morphine and nalorphine abstinence reactions with easily quantifiable and objective behavioral measures. Furthermore, the sensitivity of the method was such that evidence for an abstinence reaction could be found in rats maintained on doses of morphine as low as 1 mg/kg twice daily, ie, at doses around the minimum frequently used to assess acute effects of morphine in nontolerant rats (Pilcher and Stolerman, 1976 a,b). Such observations suggest that great care should be taken before assuming that the self-administration of opioids in low doses is not influenced by withdrawal reactions.

The experiments on naloxone-induced CTA may also significantly affect the interpretation of earlier studies on the oral self-administration of morphine (Stolerman and Kumar, 1970). It now seems possible that the behavior called "preferences" for morphine solutions could equally well be called "aversions" to tap water, the alternative source of fluid in those studies. The rats may have learned not that bitter-tasting substances were followed by the pharma-cological effects of morphine; instead, they may have acquired a CTA to tap water since on occasions when they drank it instead of the morphine solution, they would subsequently have been exposed to an increasingly intense abstinence reaction.

Presently available information does not enable a distinction to be made between the original explanation of morphine preference in terms of primary reinforcement and the new account based on CTA. The plausibility of the latter is strengthened by indications that the natural as well as the antagonist precipitated abstinence reactions may be able to support CTA (Parker and Radow, 1974). Although CTA to familiar fluids such as tap water is slow to develop, it appears eventually (Elkins, 1974; Nakajima, 1974); nobody who has worked on oral morphine intake in rats needs to be reminded that this behavior also takes a long time to develop. In the special circumstances of the morphine-preference experiments, a powerful CTA may have had a considerable but unintended influence on the amounts of drug that were self-administered. A clearer example of the need to take account of possible CTAs when conducting self-administration research can hardly be expected.

CONDITIONED TASTE AVERSIONS PRODUCED BY AMPHETAMINE

The successful development of a CTA has frequently been taken as evidence that the drug or other event acting as the unconditioned stimulus can serve an aversive function. The preceding series of experiments with naloxone was initiated with such an assumption, but Goudie (1979) has warned that merely because a drug (ie, naloxone) can be found that supports both operant avoidance/escape behavior and CTA, it does not follow that it is serving a similar stimulus function in the two cases. Indeed, as long ago as 1971, Cappell and his co-workers had shown that CTA could be induced with several psychoactive drugs which had not previously been thought to have aversive properties. These drugs were amphetamine, morphine, alcohol, and chlordiazepoxide. Supporting observations with these and other drugs many of which produced dependence in man appeared from many more laboratories and Cappell and Le Blanc (1975; 1977) provided excellent reviews.

These observations of CTA produced by agents which, far from being grossly toxic or emetic, were actually capable of supporting operant self-administration behavior by serving as positive reinforcers stimulated much of the work into a so-called "paradox;" how can the same agent both serve as a positive reinforcer and yet appear to have aversive properties? Prior to reviewing one series of attempts to answer this question, it is worth noting that other, as yet unresolved, basic questions in CTA research might have some bearing on the matter. On the one hand, CTA is most frequently categorized as a form of classical conditioning, presumably because presentations of the unconditioned stimulus are related in time to (consummatory) behavior, but are not programmed as consequences of behavior; regardless of how much behavior is elicited (or emitted?), the rat receives the same dose of drug. On the other hand, the drinking response can be treated as either an operant or a respondent and, more to the point, the amount of contact that the animal makes with the conditioned stimulus (flavor) is very much contingent on its behavior. Eliminating this contingency by directly infusing flavored solutions into the mouth weakened but did not abolish the development of CTA (Domjan and Wilson, 1972). These and related findings have been discussed more fully by Spiker (1977).

Common preconceptions about the determinants of behavior have frequently delayed acceptance of research findings; however, there are ample precedents establishing that the same event can serve either positively reinforcing or aversive functions. This seems to be the case both with common exteroceptive stimuli such as electric shock and even with narcotic antagonist drugs (Morse and Kelleher, 1977; Goldberg et al, 1971). There should be little more difficulty in accepting that, for example, amphetamine can serve superficially contrasting stimulus functions than in accepting that it can either increase or decrease the rate at which behavior is emitted according to dose, schedule-associated factors or the previous history of the organism.

Goldberg and Spealman (1982) have reported that in squirrel monkeys, infusions of nicotine can either reinforce or punish behavior depending on the circumstances surrounding their presentation. An explanation that drugs have different effects in different circumstances, while very likely correct, is inadequate with regard to CTA and self-administration because it has no predictive power unless the critical factor or factors can be identified. Thus, the robustness and reproducibility of both the reinforcing and the CTA effects of amphetamine provoked the experiments now described.

When the ability of amphetamine to produce CTA was first reported, it seemed possible that the doses used may have been too large to support self-administration behavior (Cappell and Le Blanc, 1971). Although later experiments from the same laboratory used a range of doses and still produced only CTA without any sign of a conditioned taste "preference," the conditions used were such that the appearance of any other result was very unlikely (Cappell and Le Blanc, 1973). The baseline comprised the consumption of highly palatable saccharin solutions which were presented as the only source of fluid to rats severely deprived of water. It was thought possible that different results might have been obtained if the baseline of fluid intake was decreased. D'Mello et al (1977) reinvestigated the role of dose-level in conjunction with manipulations of deprivation level, palatability of solutions, times of drug injections and presence of spatial as well as flavor stimuli.

The procedure used in these studies involved two-flavor discriminations similar to those described above in connection with the experiments on naloxone-induced CTA. The period of access to flavored solutions was reduced to 15 min in order to shorten the delay between contact with the flavor and onset of drug effect. The lowest dose of amphetamine which produced statistically significant CTA was 0.1 mg/kg, whereas when the dose of amphetamine was increased to 3.2 mg/kg, intake of the amphetamine-paired flavor was almost completely suppressed after only a single flavor-amphetamine pairing (Booth et al, 1977). These dose-response relations were broadly consistent with those found in other laboratories (Cappell and Le Blanc, 1973; Nathan and Vogel, 1975).

Neither increasing nor decreasing the interval between presentation of the flavor and injection of amphetamine (1 mg/kg), nor decreasing the baseline amounts of fluid intake altered the final degree of CTA developed after four flavor-amphetamine pairings (D'Mello et al, 1977). Decreases in dose to as low as 0.01 mg/kg, even when combined with reductions in baseline drinking levels, failed to enhance the intake of amphetamine-paired flavors; either there was a weak CTA, or if the dose was too small, there was no effect at all. An amphetamine-produced taste "preference" cannot be obtained simply by manipulating parameters of the situation where it produces CTA.

Exteroceptive stimuli paired with reinforcing drug injections can also maintain behavior (Goldberg et al, 1975). Thus, it may be supposed that during drug self-administration experiments, animals may be required to orientate themselves to a particular position in their immediate environment, such as that where the response device may be found. D'Mello et al (1977) examined the role of spatial cues by ensuring that in some rats, the flavored solutions followed by drug injections were always placed on the same side of the cage, whereas the saline-paired flavored solution was always placed on the other side of the cage. Thus, the possibility of increased drinking in places where drinking had previously been followed by amphetamine injections was pitted against the acquisition of the amphetamine CTA. However, CTA developed to about the same extent regardless of whether the rats were presented with flavor cues only or with flavor and possible competing spatial cues. Similar findings have been reported by Martin and Ellinwood (1974).

The negative result of the preceding experiment was used to argue against a role for stimulus modality as a factor determining whether amphetamine maintains or suppresses behavior, but it was not conclusive. Variables which may have contributed to the negative finding include differences in the saliency of the flavor and spatial cues, and the initial spatial preferences of the animals prior to conditioning, which may have been too strong to be shifted. Reicher and Holman (1977) presented evidence in favor of stimulus modality as a determining factor, Rats were injected with amphetamine (1.4 mg/kg) and were then confined in one side of a shuttle box in the presence of a flavored solution and of distinctive visual and tactual cues. Subsequently, the rats showed on extremely weak preference for the side of the box associated with amphetamine over the side associated with saline, but would not drink the amphetamine-paired solution.

In most self-administration experiments, amphetamine has been taken intravenously, whereas in CTA studies the intraperitoneal route has probably been the most widely used. However, both phenomena have been demonstrated with several routes and there is presently no evidence that simply injecting a drug intraperitoneally instead of intravenously is sufficient to reverse its effects in these experiments. Specifically, Wise et al (1976) and Coussens (1974) have reported on CTA produced by amphetamine administered intravenously. Another possibly relevant factor relates to the frequency of dosing; self-administration typically occurs over many sessions and could perhaps be attributed to chronic effects of drugs, whereas in many cases CTA occurs after an acute administration. This argument is weakened by observations of reinforcing effects of amphetamine within single sessions of self-administration in a very high proportion of the rats tested (eg, Davis and Smith, 1973; 1975), although the weight that can be attached to evidence from these experiments is limited by the narrow range of environmental conditions, the lack of dose-response information, and the general desirability of independent replications. It has not yet proved possible to produce enhanced intakes of flavored solutions after chronic administration of drugs such as amphetamine, although there is a large literature detailing attenuations of CTA after previous exposure to drugs (eg, Cappell and Le Blanc, 1975; Goudie et al, 1976).

It has sometimes been suggested that an animal's control of the rate at which stimuli are received may be important in determining their reinforcing value. Behavior was maintained by termination of the same parameters and temporal pattern of stimuli that themselves maintained intracranial self-stimulation behavior (Steiner et al, 1969), although the negative reinforcing effects seemed less powerful than the more frequently studied positive reinforcement. This principle may also be relevant to drug self-administration during which an animal typically has considerable control over the frequency of drug intake, which is not the case during CTA experiments where a single dose is given by the experimenter at a predetermined time (Vogel and Nathan, 1975).

The study of Stolerman et al (1971) provides an instance where rats had control over the amounts and temporal patterning of amphetamine intake, and yet the drug seemed to have aversive effects. The procedures in this study were similar to those used successfully for developing the preferential intake of morphine solutions. Initially, the rats consumed approximately equal amounts of dilute amphetamine solutions and water. Over successive choice tests, the intake of the drug solution was suppressed in a concentration-related manner. This was not simply due to a hypodipsic effect of the drug since the consumption of the plain water which was also available remained high. It was suggested that the solutions of amphetamine were rejected because the drug had an aversive pharmacological effect. If the drug solution was unpalatable, it should have been rejected on the first choice trial, which was not the case, and masking the taste should have increased intake. In fact, adding saccharin enhanced the rate at which the aversion developed, presumably because this made the drug solutions more easily discriminable from water (Hill and Powell, 1976). Other experiments have amply confirmed the apparently aversive effects of amphetamine added to rats' food or water

(Le Magnen, 1969; Carey, 1973a; Panksepp and Booth, 1973; Glick, 1973). Experiments of this type seem to demonstrate nothing more or less than CTA produced by orally self-administered amphetamine.

There are also a number of studies where stimuli paired with programmed administrations of drugs acquired positively reinforcing properties (Davis and Smith, 1973; Marcus et al, 1976; Numan et al, 1976). The weight that can be given to these comparisons is limited by the absence of a systematic study with amphetamine similar to that carried out with electric shock; visual stimuli paired with programmed shocks acquired aversive properties, but the same visual stimuli paired with the same number and temporal pattern of response-produced shocks did not become aversive (Orme-Johnson and Yarczower, 1974). Although none of the experiments reported to date seem to have compared directly the effects of programmed with self-administered amphetamine, they all militate against this factor as critical for the production of CTA.

Finally, attention was given to the role of response variables since the preceding considerations tended to exclude most of the other obvious factors. These experiments are described next and, while also failing to resolve "the paradox", they do show how flavor-drug pairings can have a very powerful influence on operant behavior and they may have considerable heuristic value.

INFLUENCE OF CONDITIONED TASTE AVERSIONS ON OPERANT BEHAVIOR

The type of response required from the rat is one of the many variables which may be relevant to the multiple stimulus properties of amphetamine; CTA involves drinking but self-administration typically requires bar-pressing. Seligman and Hager (1972) were among those who argued that different classes of response were conditioned most rapidly by different classes of consequences; it was suggested that flavor-drug pairings would exert less effect on an "arbitrary" operant such as bar-pressing than on a "naturalistic" consummatory response such as drinking. However, little evidence was cited to suggest that flavors were inherently unable to influence schedule-controlled behavior in ways resembling the more frequently studied auditory or visual stimuli. The experimental techniques used in CTA research generally involved only a limited range of standardized measurements. Usually, only aspects of the gross intake of food or water were assessed and much less was known about possible changes in other types of behavior after encounters with drug-paired flavors (Best et al, 1971).

The effects of flavor-amphetamine pairings were examined on bar-pressing for liquid reinforcers delivered on fixed ratio and fixed interval schedules. In the first of these experiments, rats were trained to press a bar for water delivered on a fixed ratio 40 schedule (FR 40). For certain sessions in the next stage of the experiment, flavored solutions were presented in the dipper cup instead of distilled water. At the end of each such session, the rats were injected with either amphetamine (1 mg/kg) or saline, and were then returned to their home cages. The two flavored solutions were presented alternately until each rat had been presented with each flavor on four occasions over a period of several weeks. On days between those on which flavored solutions were presented, the rats responded for distilled water; no injections were given (Stolerman and D'Mello, 1978a).

In some of the rats, lemon-flavored water was repeatedly paired with saline and chicken-flavored water with amphetamine. On the first occasion that each flavored solution was presented, responding did not differ greatly from that for the distilled water which was available previously. Responding for the lemon-flavored water remained reasonably stable throughout the experiment. After only a single pairing of chicken flavored water with amphetamine, responding was disrupted on the next occasion that the chicken flavor was presented. An even more marked disruption of responding was seen after further flavor-amphetamine pairings, culminating in total suppression after a single "reinforcer" in the fifth session where chicken flavored-water was presented.

The results just described could merely have been due to an unconditioned effect of chicken flavored water, although the trend across sessions made this unlikely. However, in some rats, the flavor-injection pairings were reversed; in these animals suppression of responding developed to lemon flavor, whereas responding for chicken flavor remained reasonably stable.

Similar experiments were carried out with rats which were initially stabilized on a fixed interval 1 min schedule of water reinforcement (FI 1). Responding for whichever flavor was paired with amphetamine (1 mg/kg) was disrupted after a single drug administration; responding for the control flavor remained stable. The disruptive effects became more marked after repeated flavor-amphetamine pairings (D'Mello and Stolerman, 1978).

After flavor-amphetamine pairings, both bar-pressing for and the mean amounts consumed of the flavored liquids were greatly reduced. The reductions in fluid intake was brought about partly by the presentation of fewer reinforcers and partly by a reduced consumption of the reinforcers which were obtained. The temporal pattern of responding was assessed by means of the index of curvature described by Fry et al (1960). Amphetamine-paired flavors decreased the value of the index, but this was mainly attributed to the very marked reductions in the total numbers of responses. Responding was irregular throughout the intervals, but at no time was its rate increased by amphetamine-paired flavors.

Amphetamine (1 mg/kg) was injected 5 min before sessions of responding for distilled water at a later stage of these experiments. This dose of the drug reduced the total numbers of responses emitted by the rats on the FR 40 schedule without influencing total responses or the amounts of water consumed under the FI 1 schedule. However, the temporal pattern of FI responding was disrupted since the drug increased the numbers of responses early in the intervals and decreased the numbers of responses late in the intervals (D'Mello and Stolerman, 1978). These well-known, schedule-associated effects of amphetamine confirmed the adequacy of the schedule manipulations.

It was concluded that flavor-amphetamine pairings could have a very powerful influence on operant behavior and that this was worthy of more intensive study, albeit that suppression of the consummatory response may have mediated the effect. Insofar as the results involved only one dose of amphetamine and two schedules of reinforcement, they were considered as preliminary, but it was difficult in the face of such data to attribute the contrasting reinforcing and aversive properties of amphetamine merely to the classes of responses required by the experimental procedures. The effects of the amphetamine-paired flavors were not schedule-dependent and were much greater than those of omitting the primary water reinforcement throughout the session. The conditioned effects of the flavors were therefore different from the effects of either the unconditioned stimulus (amphetamine) or of an extinction procedure. Glowa and Barrett (1983) have extended these findings by showing that post-session injections of amphetamine paired with visual stimuli can suppress responding in pigeons. There is a very striking contrast between these findings and those where single, post-session injections of drugs maintain responding of monkeys on second-order schedules (Goldberg et al, 1975; Katz, 1979). Analogous positive reinforcing effects of post-session injections in rats seem not to have been reported, but might provide a basis for further studies of variables affecting the appearance of CTA.

The experiments reviewed up to now have tended to exclude as critical factors drug dose, route of administration, acute versus chronic dosing, baseline amounts of behavior, stimulus modality and response variables. In some cases the evidence was strong, in others it was weak and derived from experiments originally carried out for other reasons. This was particularly the case because the problem seems largely one of acquisition of behavior, which has been of secondary concern in many studies of drug self-administration. Nevertheless, the research was fast approaching an impasse where every possible factor seemed to have been excluded and it was decided to adopt a more pharmacological approach in a further attempt to resolve the "paradox."

A PHARMACOLOGICAL APPROACH TO
CONDITIONED TASTE AVERSION

Many hypotheses have been presented as to what actions of drugs produce CTA, but no mechanism has been generally agreed. In early work, radiation or drugs with obvious toxic effects were used, and despite the multiple effects which such treatments had, it was assumed that toxicity, nausea, gastrointestinal distress, or illness was responsible for the CTA. These ideas received little experimental testing until Coil et al (1978) reported that pretreatment with antiemetic agents reduced the suppression of CTA produced by lithium, but attempts to replicate these observations have not yet been successful (Goudie et al, 1982; Rabin and Hunt, 1983). In general, notions such as distress or illness proved difficult to assess and the potency of drugs in producing such effects was not found to correlate with their potency in CTA (reviewed by Braveman, 1977; Goudie, 1979). The CTA produced by nutrient substances or by very low doses of psychoactive drugs such as amphetamine was also difficult to explain as solely due to toxicity (Cappell and Le Blanc, 1975; Deutsch et al, 1976).

The aim of the experiments described here was to determine the relative potencies of (+)-amphetamine and some related compounds. It was known from earlier work that there were differences between the profiles of action of these substances, and it was hoped that effects such as anorexia, or actions on particular neurochemical systems, could be correlated with potency in producing CTA. Studies with congeners of amphetamine had been reported previously, but comparisons between different drugs can be misleading unless a range of doses of each substance is studied with a standardized procedure.

The results from this series of experiments showed that it was feasible to use a standardized, discriminative CTA procedure to examine differences in potency between different amphetamines (Booth et al, 1977). Even small groups of rats, counterbalanced for flavor-injection pairings and injection sequences, gave reliable results. Indeed, the method was sensitive enough to give results with (+)- and (−)-amphetamine which suggested that the relative effectiveness of drugs may be dependent on time-related factors; delayed injections differentiated between the isomers whereas low doses failed to do so. The study also showed that in CTA, p-chloromethamphetamine was significantly more potent than the parent compound, methamphetamine. These two substances had previously been found to be approximately equipotent as anorexigenic agents in rats, but p-chloromethamphetamine had only about one tenth the potency of methamphetamine in facilitating conditioned avoidance behavior (Cox and Maickel, 1972).

It was found that agents potent in producing CTA may be either powerful (amphetamine, methamphetamine) or weak (fenfluramine, p-chloromethamphetamine) behavioral stimulants. Furthermore, cocaine, a powerful stimulant, was weak in CTA. Firstly, therefore, it appeared that the potency of amphetamine congeners in producing CTA was unrelated to their stimulant potency. Secondly, the CTA produced by the halogen-substituted derivatives p-chloromethamphetamine and fenfluramine was at least as great as that of the unsubstituted parent compounds; CTA potency could not be correlated with the differential activity of these drugs on catecholamine and serotonin mechanisms. Thirdly, the CTA effect of amphetamine was largely central since para-hydroxylation greatly reduced conditioning, but this conclusion has been challenged recently (Greenshaw and Buresova, 1982). *In vitro* experiments have indicated little difference between the effects of (+)-amphetamine and p-hydroxyamphetamine on aminergic mechanisms, but the more polar hydroxy-derivative penetrates poorly to the brain. This conclusion about the site of action has been supported by a number of other studies discussed by Lorden et al (1980). Finally, the most effective agents in producing CTA seemed to have in common a powerful anorexigenic effect and a long duration of action. The significance of these two factors was investigated in turn.

The conditioned anorexia hypothesis attempts to account for CTA as classical conditioning of the anorexigenic or hypodipsic effects of drugs to the flavor stimuli (Le Magnen, 1969; Carey and Goodall, 1974). Such conditioning would be expected to decrease the intake of flavored solutions, thus producing the effect typically seen in CTA experiments. The idea was attractive since it related CTA to a known behavioral effect and if correct, it would have helped to explain how many self-administered drugs appeared to have aversive properties in CTA procedures; if CTA was essentially a complex way for assessing anorexigenic activity, then its validity as a measure of aversiveness would have been undermined. However, events soon indicated that this rather radical reinterpretation of CTA was unnecessary.

Doses of X-radiation which induced CTA did not produce hypodipsia (Garcia et al, 1972; Carroll and Smith, 1974), whereas chlordiazepoxide, a drug which frequently increases food intake, also produced clear CTA (Cappell and Le Blanc, 1975). Doses of lithium, ammonium sulphate, arginine, and glucose which produced similar degrees of anorexia produced varying intensities of CTA (Martin and Storlien, 1976). All these findings argued against the conditioned anorexia hypothesis, but experiments with amphetamines seemed to support it. Carey and Goodall (1974) reported that the relative potencies of (+)- and (−)-amphetamine were similar in CTA and hypodipsia experiments. The studies by Booth et al (1977) also consistently suggested a possible correlation between potencies in these two procedures. Although conditioned anorexia seemed not to be viable as an account of CTA in general, it might have been tenable with regard to CTA produced by amphetamine, a noted and indeed prototypical anorexigenic drug. However, Booth et al (1977) had to rely on estimates of anorexigenic activity based on studies from other laboratories and comparisons with their own work on CTA were difficult for several reasons, each one of which might have influenced relative potencies. It was therefore necessary to compare the results of the CTA studies with assessments of hypodipsia carried out under similar conditions in the same laboratory (Stolerman and D'Mello, 1978b).

The results confirmed that the hypodipsic potency of (+)-amphetamine was at least three times that of (−)-amphetamine. Under very similar conditions, and in rats of the same sex, strain and weight, the two isomers were essentially equipotent in CTA (potency ratio = 1.2:1). Cox and Maickel (1972) found little difference between the anorexigenic potencies of methamphetamine and p-chloromethamphetamine, and the finding that the hypodipsic potencies of these drugs were similar (1.1:1) was therefore not surprising. Nevertheless, p-chloromethamphetamine was at least twice as potent as methamphetamine in CTA. In summary, drugs which are equipotent in CTA can differ in hypodipsic potency, and drugs with similar hypodipsic potencies can differ in CTA. Fenfluramine also had less than half the hypodipsic potency of (+)-amphetamine, but was at least equipotent in CTA. In a dose of 2 mg/kg, fenfluramine produced very strong CTA after only a single flavor-injection pairing, whereas this dose of the drug was totally lacking in hypodipsic activity. The various dissociations between hypodipsic and CTA potencies were incompatible with the conditioned anorexia hypothesis of amphetamine-induced CTA.

Other lines of research have also yielded evidence which appears inconsistent with the conditioned anorexia hypothesis of amphetamine CTA. Pretreatment with α-methyl-p-tyrosine can differentiate the responses to amphetamine and to amphetamine-paired flavors (Carey, 1973b). The effects of presenting flavored solutions previously paired with amphetamine (1 mg/kg) were uniformly depressant on FR 40 and FI 1 responding, whereas the same dose of amphetamine produced the well-known, rate-dependent effects (see above). Thus, the conditioned response to the flavored solutions differed from the response to the drug both in the studies where the solutions were freely available for drinking and in the studies where they were presented on intermittent schedules. Since conditioned anorexia did not seem to account for CTA produced by amphetamine, attention was then focussed on the growing body of evidence that the duration of drug action was a critical factor.

The results from several laboratories consistently implied that the longer the duration of action of a drug, the more effective it was likely to be in producing CTA (Cappell and Le Blanc, 1975; 1977; Goudie et al, 1978; Booth et al, 1977). Testa and Ternes (1977) provided a theoretical basis for such ideas. Cocaine, a short-acting drug, was of low potency whereas the long-acting halogen-substituted amphetamines such as fenfluramine and p-chloromethamphetamine were very potent in CTA. The conclusions that could be reached from this work were limited because, in most cases, the drugs between which comparisons were made differed in several respects in addition to duration of action. Furthermore, pretreatment with the metabolic inhibitor SKF-525A increased the effectiveness of amphetamine but not that of cocaine (Goudie and Thornton, 1977; Goudie, 1980). In one experiment, it was shown that a 4-hr inhalation of nitrous oxide produced greater CTA than a 30-min inhalation (Goudie and Dickens, 1978).

The recent development of long-acting analogues of cocaine and apomorphine provided an opportunity for reassessing the role of duration of drug action in CTA (D'Mello et al, 1981). It was known that some behavioral and neurochemical effects of the cocaine analogue Win 35,428 were qualitatively similar to those of cocaine, but it had a considerably longer duration of action and was more potent as a central stimulant (Spealman et al, 1977; Heikkila et al, 1979). Diisobutyrylapomorphine (DBA) had prolonged apomorphine-like behavioral effects but was similar in potency to apomorphine (Baldessarini et al, 1976; 1977). Comparisons of cocaine with Win 35,428 and of apomorphine with DBA seemed likely to provide more critical tests of the role of duration of action in CTA than, for example, the comparison of cocaine with amphetamine. For these new comparisons to be meaningful, it was necessary to know the relative potencies of the drugs in a standard behavioral procedure in the relevant species. For this reason the compounds were studied on behavior maintained by a fixed ratio schedule as well as in CTA.

In sufficient doses, all the drugs produced CTA and in general, the greater the dose, the more marked was the CTA. Cocaine produced significant CTA only at 100 μmol/kg, the largest dose tested, whereas the lowest effective dose of Win 35,428 was 1.8 μmol/kg. Apomorphine and DBA produced CTA at 0.32 μmol/kg (the lowest dose tested) and at all higher doses. In the study of operant behavior, the key-press responding of rats was maintained at high steady rates by a fixed ratio 30 schedule of food reinforcement. All the drugs reduced response rates in a dose-related manner and except for cocaine, the largest doses used almost completely suppressed responding. Studies of time-effect relations with cocaine and Win 35,428 on the FR 30 schedule confirmed the approximately tripled duration of action of the analogue. Win 35,428 was also much more potent than cocaine, whereas apomorphine and DBA did not differ from each other in potency.

Two potency ratios were derived for cocaine and Win 35,428, one based on the studies of CTA (ratio of 35:1) and the other on the studies of FR 30 responding (ratio of 41:1). Clearly, these potency ratios agreed well with each other. There was also close agreement between potency ratios for apomorphine and DBA derived from the studies of CTA and FR 30 responding (ratios of 1.0:1 and 1.1:1 respectively).

Since the potency ratios for cocaine and apomorphine relative to their long-acting analogues Win 35,428 and DBA were essentially the same in the CTA and the FR 30 procedures, it was suggested that even marked increases in duration of action do not necessarily have a specific effect on potency in CTA. Goudie and Dickins (1978) have relied upon temporal factors to explain why many drugs with positively reinforcing effects can also produce CTA, but such accounts seem to need revision if not rejection since none of the experiments reported to date has established unequivocally that potency in CTA is correlated with duration of action.

SUMMARY AND CONCLUSIONS

The experiments discussed in the preceding sections of this article provided several examples of ways in which the conditioning of taste aversions, either intentionally or accidentally, might have influenced drug-taking behavior. Although considerable progress has been made in producing sustained high levels of oral intake of opioid drugs, the possibility that unintended CTA might control this behavior in some circumstances has not been much discussed; the demonstrations of clear CTA produced by the morphine abstinence reaction suggests that such possibilities deserve serious consideration. Indeed, CTA seemed to provide a particularly sensitive behavioral marker for precipitated withdrawal signs with opioids, suggesting that it might also have potential in similar applications with other classes of drugs where abstinence phenomena are much harder to identify by methods used until now. It has been also shown that the oral intake of opioids can be suppressed by CTA produced to their tastes by a variety of agents, including but not limited to naloxone (Fernandez and Ternes, 1975; Ternes, 1975; Mumford et al, 1978). The schedule-induced consumption of drug solutions can be suppressed by taste aversion conditioning, but there is some doubt as to whether the suppression is as great as with deprivation-induced fluid intake (Corfield-Sumner and Bond, 1978; Riley et al, 1979).

Most of these studies assumed that CTA was, as its name implied, a straightforward means for assessing aversive effects of drugs. The demonstrations of CTA produced by self-administered substances provides a challenge insofar as a full analysis of the effect might yield information about aversive properties of drugs which limit their intake, perhaps even in the conventional self-administration situations. Drug-taking behavior could then be regarded as regulated by a balance between positively reinforcing and aversive drug effects (Kumar and Stolerman, 1977) and indeed, such assumptions lay behind many of the studies of amphetamine-produced CTA which were discussed earlier.

In virtually the only study of its type, Gorman et al (1978) attempted to assess directly the relations between the CTA effect of morphine and oral self-administration of the same drug. Rats were first subjected to a conventional CTA procedure with injected morphine as the unconditioned stimulus, and were then offered sweetened morphine solutions as an alternative to plain water. Rats in which the CTA was very marked subsequently self-administered only small amounts of morphine, the implication being that the CTA effects of morphine are relevant to self-administration and can limit its extent. These studies need to be replicated and developed further before any general conclusions can be reached since Gorman et al (1978) reported only a transient, strain-dependent correlation between CTA and self-administration. Furthermore, only one of the experiments controlled for stimulus generalization between the flavor cue in the CTA phase and the sweetened water in which morphine was subsequently presented; unfortunately, in just this one experiment, CTA was barely detectable.

Long series of experiments carried out in various laboratories have failed to identify any specific behavioral or pharmacological variables which might determine whether reinforcing or aversive effects of drugs predominate in a given situation. Dose level, route of administration, frequency of dosing the subjects' control over the situation, stimulus and response variables all seem to be contraindicated by one or more experiments. Although some of the evidence on these matters is inconclusive, the overall trend suggests that the wrong questions may have been asked. Instead of searching for controlling variables in the ways described, perhaps it would be worthwhile to question the interpretations of the basic datum; is the development of CTA sufficient to establish that the event serving as the unconditioned stimulus really has aversive properties? Although there is no doubt that very powerful and reproducible behavioral changes can occur in CTA studies, could the naming of the phenomenon as "conditioned taste aversion" have directed attention away from how it is best interpreted? In a review, McKearney and Barrett (1978) commented,

> Events that control behavior are necessarily presented or with-
> drawn according to a schedule, and the exact nature of this
> relation between behavior and its consequences is of inestimable
> importance in determining both ongoing behavior itself and the
> behavioral effects of drugs. Indeed, the processes of reinforcement
> and punishment cannot be conceptualized independently of
> considerations related to the scheduling of consequent events.

As Spiker (1977) has emphasized, much remains to be done before it can be claimed that the exact nature of the relations between behavior and consequences in CTA experiments has been analyzed fully.

It can now be argued that CTA produced by self-administered drugs or by drug-induced withdrawal reactions may have a very significant influence on oral drug self-administration, as illustrated above for morphine and amphetamine. It is also reasonable to suppose that these influences are not limited solely to consummatory responding, but extend also to operant behavior maintained by presentations of drug solutions. Before extrapolations can be made to other laboratory situations or to drug dependence in humans, answers to some very basic questions about CTA are still needed. Precisely which aspects of the contingencies in CTA are necessary and sufficient for the effect to occur? What characteristics are shared by the drugs which are effective in producing CTA? How far can the implication that aversive drug effects limit oral intake be extended to other self-administration situations, possibly including the intravenous paradigms, or are the CTA effects specific to particular species, stimuli and responses? Indeed (Stolerman and D'Mello, 1981) have questioned whether it is reasonable to make even the common assumption that the drugs used in CTA are serving an aversive stimulus function. The relative neglect of this whole area by behavioral pharmacologists, despite its twenty-five year history and its prominence in the psychological literature, can be traced to the very different, ethologically-orientated, theoretical positions held by most of the pioneering researchers in CTA and to the associated polemics from both groups. Elimination of these restrictive influences and further integration of the two approaches seems to be long overdue; it is obvious that CTA, regardless of whether it is best considered as classical conditioning, punishment, or conditioned suppression, can have very powerful effects, the full significance of which can only be determined by future research.

REFERENCES

Baldessarini RJ, Walton KG and Borgman RJ: Prolonged apomorphine-like behavioral effects of apomorphine esters. *Neuropharm* 15:471–478, 1976

Baldessarini RJ, Kula NS, Walton KG and Borgman RJ: Behavioral effects of apomorphine and diisobutyrylapomorphine in the mouse. *Psychopharmacol* 53:45–53, 1977

Best PJ, Best MR and Ahlers RH: Transfer of discriminated taste aversion to a leverpressing task. *Psychonomic Science* 25:281–282, 1971

Booth DA, D'Mello GD, Pilcher CWT and Stolerman IP: Comparative potencies of amphetamine, fenfluramine and related compounds in taste aversion experiments in rats. *Br J Pharmacol* 61:669–677, 1977

Braveman NS: What studies on pre-exposure to pharmacological agents tell us about the nature of the aversion-inducing agent? In: LM Barker, M Best and M Domjan (eds.), *Learning Mechanisms in Food Selection.* Waco, Texas: Baylor University Press, pp 511–530, 1977

Cappell H and Le Blanc AE: Conditioned aversion to saccharin by single administrations of mescaline and d-amphetamine. *Psychopharmacologia* 22:352–356, 1971

Cappell H and Le Blanc AE: Punishment of saccharin drinking by amphetamine in rats and its reversal by chlordiazepoxide. *J Comparative Physiol Psychol* 85:97–104, 1973

Cappell H and Le Blanc AE: Conditioned aversion by psychoactive drugs: Does it have significance for an understanding of drug dependence? *Addictive Behaviors* 1:55–64, 1975

Cappell H and Le Blanc AE: Gustatory avoidance conditioning by drugs of abuse. In: NW Milgram, L Krames and TM Alloway (eds.), *Food Aversion Learning.* New York: Plenum, pp 133–167, 1977

Carey RJ: Acquired aversion to amphetamine solutions. *Pharmacology, Biochemistry and Behavior* 1:227–229, 1973a

Carey RJ: Long-term aversion to a saccharin solution induced by repeated amphetamine injections. *Pharmacology, Biochemistry and Behavior* 1:265–270, 1973b

Carey RJ and Goodall EB: Amphetamine-induced taste aversion: A comparison of d- versus l-amphetamine. *Pharmacology, Biochemistry and Behavior* 2:325–330, 1974

Carroll ME and Smith JC: Time-course of radiation-induced taste aversion conditioning. *Physiology and Behavior* 13:809–812, 1974

Coil JD, Hankins WG, Jenden DJ and Garcia J: The attenuation of a specific cue-to-consequence association by antiemetic agents. *Psychopharmacol* 56:21–25, 1978

Corfield-Sumner PK and Bond NW: Taste aversion learning and schedule-induced alcohol consumption in rats. *Pharmacology, Biochemistry and Behavior* 9:731–733, 1978

Coussens WR: Conditioned taste aversion: Route of drug administration. In: JM Singh and H Lal (eds.), *Drug Addiction, Volume 3. Neurobiology and Influences on Behavior.* New York: Stratton Intercontinental Medical Book Co., pp. 241–248, 1974

Cox RH and Maickel RP: Comparison of anorexigenic and behavioral potency of some phenylethylamines. *J Pharmacol Exp Ther* 181:1–9, 1972

Davis WM and Smith SG: Blocking effect of α-methyltyrosine on amphetamine based reinforcement. *J Pharmacy and Pharmacology* 25:174–177, 1973

Davis WM and Smith SG: Effect of haloperidol on (+)-amphetamine self-administration. *J Pharmacy and Pharmacology* 27:540–542, 1975

Deutsch JA, Molina F and Puerto A: Conditioned taste aversion caused by palatable nontoxic nutrients. *Behav Biol* 16:161–174, 1976

D'Mello GD and Stolerman IP: Suppression of fixed-interval responding by flavour-amphetamine pairings in rats. *Pharmacology, Biochemistry and Behavior* 9: 395–398, 1978

D'Mello GD, Stolerman IP, Booth DA and Pilcher CWT: Factors influencing flavour aversions conditioned with amphetamine in rats. *Pharmacology, Biochemistry and Behavior* 7:185–190, 1977

D'Mello GD, Goldberg DM, Goldberg SR and Stolerman IP: Conditioned taste aversion and operant behavior in rats: Effects of cocaine, apomorphine and some long-acting derivatives. *J Pharmacol Exp Ther* 219:60–68, 1981

Domjan M and Wilson NE: Contribution of ingestive behaviors to taste-aversion learning in the rat. *J Comp Physiol Psychol* 80:403–412, 1972

Elkins RL: Conditioned flavor aversions to familiar tap water in rats: An adjustment with implications for aversion therapy treatment of alcoholism and obesity. *J Abnormal Psychology* 83:411–417, 1974

Fernandez B and Ternes JW: Conditioned aversion to morphine with lithium chloride in morphine-dependent rats. *Bull Psychonomic Soc* 5:331–332, 1975

Fry W, Kelleher RT and Cook L: A mathematical index of performance on fixed-interval schedules of reinforcement. *Journal of the Experimental Analysis of Behavior* 3:193–199, 1960

Garcia J and Ervin FR: Gustatory-visceral and telereceptor-cutaneous conditioning – adaptation in internal and external milieus. *Communications in Behavioral Biology* Part A, 1:389–415, 1968

Garcia J, McGowan BK and Green KF: Biological constraints on conditioning. In: AH Black and WF Prokasy (eds.), *Classical Conditioning II: Current Research and Theory*. New York: Appleton-Century-Crofts, pp 3–27, 1972

Glick SD: Impaired tolerance to the effects of oral amphetamine intake in rats with frontal cortex ablations. *Psychopharmacologia* 28:363–371, 1973

Glowa JR and Barrett JE: Response suppression by visual stimuli paired with post-session *d*-amphetamine injections in the pigeon. *J Exp Anal Behav* 39:165–173, 1983

Goldberg SR and Spealman RD: Maintenance and suppression of behavior by intravenous nicotine injections in squirrel monkeys. *Fed Proc* 41:216–220, 1982

Goldberg SR, Hoffmeister F, Schlichting U and Wuttke W: Aversive properties of nalorphine in morphine-dependent rhesus monkeys. *J Pharmacol Exp Ther* 179:268–276, 1971

Goldberg SR, Kelleher RT and Morse WH: Second-order schedules of drug injection. *Fed Proc* 34:1771–1776, 1975

Gorman JE, De Obaldia RN, Scott RC and Reid LD: Morphine injections in the taste aversion paradigm: Extent of aversions and readiness to consume sweetened morphine solutions. *Physiological Psychology* 6:101–109, 1978

Goudie AJ: Aversive stimulus properties of drugs. *Neuropharmacol* 18:971–979, 1979

Goudie AJ: Aversive stimulus properties of cocaine following inhibition of hepatic enzymes. *IRCS Medical Science* 8:58–59, 1980

Goudie AJ and Dickins DW: Nitrous oxide-induced conditioned taste aversions in rats: The role of duration of drug exposure and its relation to the taste aversion-self-administration "paradox." *Pharmacology, Biochemistry and Behavior* 9:587–592, 1978

Goudie AJ and Thornton EW: Role of drug metabolism in the aversive properties of d-amphetamine. *IRCS Medical Science* 5:93, 1977

Goudie AJ, Thornton EW and Wheeler TJ: Drug pretreatment effects in drug induced taste aversions; effects of dose and duration of pretreatment. *Pharmacology, Biochemistry and Behavior* 4:629–633, 1976

Goudie AJ, Dickins DW and Thornton EW: Cocaine-induced conditioned taste aversion in rats. *Pharmacology, Biochemistry and Behavior* 8:757–761, 1978

Goudie AJ, Stolerman IP, Demellweek C and D'Mello GD: Does conditioned nausea mediate drug-induced conditioned taste aversion? *Psychopharmacology* 78:277–281, 1982

Greenshaw AJ and Burésova O: Learned taste aversion to saccharin following intra-ventricular or intraperitoneal administration of d,l-amphetamine. *Pharmacol Biochem Behav* 17:1129-1133, 1982

Heikkila RE, Cabbat FS, Manzino L and Duvoisin RC: Rotational behavior induced by cocaine analogs in rats with unilateral 6-hydroxydopamine lesions of the substantia nigra: Dependence upon dopamine uptake inhibition. *J Pharmacol Exp Ther* 211:189-194, 1979

Hill SY and Powell BJ: Acquired preference for morphine but not *d*-amphetamine as a result of saccharine adulteration. *Psychopharmacol* 50:309-312, 1976

Katz JL: A comparison of responding maintained under second-order schedules of intramuscular cocaine injection or food presentation in squirrel monkeys. *Journal of the Experimental Analysis of Behavior* 32:419-431, 1979

Kumar R and Stolerman IP: Experimental and clinical aspects of drug dependence. In: LL Iversen, SD Iversen and SH Snyder (eds.), *Handbook of Psychopharmacology, Volume 7.* New York: Plenum, pp 321-367, 1977

Le Magnen J: Peripheral and systemic actions of food in the caloric regulation of intake. *Ann NY Acad Sci* 157:1126-1156, 1969

Lorden JF, Callahan M and Dawson R: Depletion of central catecholamines alters amphetamine- and fenfluramine-induced taste aversions in the rat. *J Comp Physiol Psychol* 94:99-114, 1980

Marcus R, Carnathan G, Meyer RE and Cochin J: Morphine-based secondary reinforce-ment: Effects of different doses of naloxone. *Psychopharmacology* 48:247-250, 1976

Martin GM and Storlien LH: Anorexia and conditioned taste aversions in the rat. *Learning and Motivation* 7:274-282, 1976

Martin JC and Ellinwood EH: Conditioned aversion in spatial paradigms following methamphetamine injection. *Psychopharmacologia* 36:323-335, 1974

McKearney JW and Barrett JE: Schedule-controlled behavior and the effects of drugs. In: DE Blackman and DJ Sanger (eds.), *Contemporary Research in Behavioral Pharmacology.* New York: Plenum, pp 1-68, 1978

Morse WH and Kelleher RT: Determinants of reinforcement and punishment. In: WK Honig and JER Staddon (eds.), *Handbook of Operant Behavior.* New Jersey: Prentice-Hall, pp 174-200, 1977

Mumford L, Teixeira AR and Kumar R: Resistance of morphine-seeking behaviour in rats to pharmacological and behavioural "treatments." *Nature* 272:167-168, 1978

Nakajima S: Conditioned aversion of water produced by cycloheximide injection. *Physiological Psychology* 2:484-486, 1974

Nathan BA and Vogel JR: Taste aversions induced by d-amphetamine: Dose-response relationship. *Bulletin of the Psychonomic Society* 6:287-288, 1975

Numan R, Banerjee U, Smith N and Lal H: Secondary reinforcement property of a stimulus paired with morphine administration in the rat. *Pharmacology, Biochemistry and Behavior* 5:395-399, 1976

Orme-Johnson DW and Yarczower M: Conditioned suppression, punishment and aversion. *Journal of the Experimental Analysis of Behavior* 21:57-74, 1974

Panksepp J and Booth DA: Tolerance in the depression of intake when amphetamine is added to the rat's food. *Psychopharmacologia* 29:45-54, 1973

Parker LF and Radow BL: Morphine-like physical dependence: A pharmacologic method for drug assessment using the rat. *Pharmacology, Biochemistry and Behavior* 2:613–618, 1974

Pilcher CWT and Stolerman IP: Conditioned flavor aversions for assessing precipitated morphine abstinence in rats. *Pharmacology, Biochemistry and Behavior* 4:159–163, 1976a

Pilcher CWT and Stolerman IP: Recent approaches to assessing opiate dependence in rats. In: HW Kosterlitz (ed.), *Opiates and Endogenous Opioid Peptides.* Amsterdam: Elsevier/North Holland, pp 327–334, 1976b

Rabin BM and Hunt WA: Effects of antiemetics on the acquisition and recall of radiation- and lithium chloride-induced conditioned taste aversions. *Pharmacol Biochem Behav* 18:629–635, 1983

Reicher MA and Holman EW: Location preference and flavor aversion reinforced by amphetamine in rats. *Animal Learning and Behavior* 5:343–346, 1977

Revusky S and Garcia J: Learned association over long delays. In: GH Bower (ed.), *The Psychology of Learning and Motivation: Advances in Research and Theory.* New York: Academic Press, pp 1–84, 1970

Riley AL, Lotter EC and Kulkosky PJ: The effects of conditioned taste aversions on the acquisition and maintenance of schedule-induced polydipsia. *Animal Learning and Behavior* 7:3–12, 1979

Seligman MEP and Hager JL: *Biological Boundaries of Learning.* New York: Appleton-Century-Crofts, 1972

Spealman RD, Goldberg SR, Kelleher RT, Goldberg DM and Charlton JP: Some effects of cocaine and two cocaine analogs on schedule-controlled behavior of squirrel monkeys. *J Pharmacol Exp Ther* 202:500–509, 1977

Spiker VA: Taste aversion: A procedural analysis and an alternative paradigmatic classification. *The Psychological Record* 27:753–769, 1977

Steiner SS, Beer B and Shaffer MM: Escape from self-produced rates of brain stimulation. *Science* 163:90–91, 1969

Stolerman IP and D'Mello GD: Amphetamine-induced taste aversion demonstrated with operant behaviour. *Pharmacology, Biochemistry and Behavior* 8:107–111, 1978a

Stolerman IP and D'Mello GD: Oral self-administration and the relevance of conditioned taste aversion. In: T Thompson, PB Dews and WA McKim (eds.), *Advances in Behavioral Pharmacology 3.* New York: Academic Press, 1981 pp 169–214

Stolerman IP and Kumar R: Preferences for morphine in rats: Validation of an experimental model of dependence. *Psychopharmacologia* 17:137–150, 1970

Stolerman IP, Kumar R and Steinberg H: Development of morphine dependence in rats; lack of effect of previous ingestion of other drugs. *Psychopharmacologia* 20:321–336, 1971

Ternes JW: Conditioned aversion to morphine with naloxone. *Bull Psychonomic Society* 5:292–294, 1975

Testa TJ and Ternes JW: Specificity of conditioning mechanisms in the modification of food preferences. In: LM Barker, MR Best and M Domjan (eds.), *Learning Mechanisms in Food Selection.* Waco, Texas: Baylor University Press, pp 229–253, 1977

Vogel JR and Nathan BA: Learned taste aversions induced by hypnotic drugs. *Pharmacology, Biochemistry and Behavior* 3:189–194, 1975

Wise RA, Yokel RA and deWit H: Both positive reinforcement and conditioned aversion from amphetamine and from apomorphine in rats. *Science* 191:1273–1275, 1976

5

Behavior in Excess:
An Examination of the Volitional Disorders

S. JOSEPH MULÉ

EXAMINATION OF THE DISORDERS

In viewing behavior as excessive, we might readily ask by what means or standard does one judge behavior as abnormal or deviant? The direct simple approach would be to consult the American Psychiatric Association's *Manual of Mental Disorders* (DSM-III). A more pragmatic approach would be simply to determine whether the behavior is harmful to the individual (deleterious medical consequences), to society (violence, stealing, impaired driving, financial dependency) or a combination of both. Once a consensus is achieved then the object of the exaggerated behavior (ie, the volitional disorder itself) may be examined (Table 1). The question is what factors or forces control the chosen excessive behavior (drugs, food, gambling, sex, work, etc.)? Does environment, socioeconomic status, position, education, and genetics contribute to the disorder engaged? Is the choice of activity solely conscious or does the unconscious play a role? However chosen, it certainly appears that the individual does not normally "decide" to become drug dependent or alcoholic or obese, etc, but in all probability over time and through continued reinforcement falls into the excess pattern which culminates in, at the very least, a psychic dependency.

The question is of course whether a commonality of processes exists between the various forms of excessive behavior (Table 2). If so, what are the shared properties and characteristics (etiological, biological, sociological, psychological) of the various volitional disorders (Table 3)? If a common thread or denominator runs through the affected individuals, then one might expect as commonplace the substitution of one substance for another (eg,

Table 1. Volitional Disorders

I. *Drugs*
   A. Opiates
   B. Sedatives, Hypnotics, Tranquilizers
   C. Psychomotor Stimulants
   D. Hallucinogens
   E. Alcohol
   F. Marijuana
   G. Tobacco
   H. Caffeine

II. *Non-Drugs*
   A. Overeating and obesity
   B. Anorexia nervosa
   C. Nymphomania and Satyriasis
   D. Excessive work
   E. Gambling
   F. Television
   G. Excessive sports

Table 2. Commonalities

1. Multiple substance use or behavioral activity
2. Unconcerned about well being
3. Hustling
4. Less than optimum state of arousal normally
5. Ease of obtaining reinforcement—no hassle
6. Genetics
7. Nutrition—diet
8. Effects—short-term or long-term
9. Culture
10. Social setting—environment
11. Enjoy altered state of consciousness

Table 3. Characteristics of Volitional Disorders

A. Etiological
B. Psychological
C. Biochemical
D. Pharmacological
E. Economical
F. Sociological

methadone for heroin), or the excessive use reliance or dependence on several substances at the same time (heroin, alcohol, tobacco, marihuana, stimulants), or one behavioral disorder for another (overeating for smoking), or involvement in a plethora of overactive behaviors in the realms of drinking, eating, smoking, sex, gambling, etc, simultaneously. If such a commonality between behavior patterns in fact does occur, then a general theory might identify and provide a cogent explanation for the underlying cause of the exaggerated behaviors. Thus, the *volitional disorders* may simply be the end result of a conflict between internal and external forces (Table 4); such as: (a) predisposition (genetic, nutrition, sociocultural, socioeconomic, temperament); (b) environment (the external surroundings may enhance or inhibit the predisposing forces); (c) fortifications (behavior is reinforced through repetition and interactions of a pharmacological, biochemical, psychological or sociological nature); (d) tolerance (continued interaction of the substance or exaggerated behavior with the physiological system); (e) physiochemical adjustment (homeostatic mechanisms require continued substance use or excessive activity to prevent a negative adjustment in the system); (f) abstinence (withdrawal symptoms occur when the level of substance use or activity is insufficient to maintain the dependent state); (g) hypophoria (negative feeling states relieved by excessive behavior).

An example of how the excessive behavior occurs might be provided by the socioeconomically deprived ghetto youngster who becomes involved with heroin use through peer pressure and finds such use an acceptable means of alleviating negative personal feelings (anxiety, insecurity, hostility, frustration) allowing him to "feel good" about himself and his environment. On the other hand a middle class Irish Catholic white male may resort to excessive alcohol use as the preferred vehicle for alleviating his hypophoric state and thus capture the same "feel good" aura. It is of course not difficult to draw similar profiles for overeaters, excessive smokers, anorexics, compulsive gamblers, compulsive and excessive sport activists, overworkers, and television addicts. It the etiology of the volitional disorders (Table 5) can be identified irrespective of the chosen excessive behavior, then an effective therapeutic remedy can be found. Hopefully, a basic therapeutic modality might unfold allowing for a direct attack at the psychic source of the disorder, leading to an extinction of the outward exaggerated behavioral expression. The modality must also be capable of altering or assisting in correcting the physiological as well as the socioeconomic correlates of the disorder.

It is worthwhile to comment at this point on the various components which may characterize the volitional disorders (Table 6). These appear to be an illusionary conception of an exalted superior state (grandiosity). Hypophoria, compulsivity, obsession, and loss of control over one's behavior; also depression, insecurity, frustration and anxiety may be present.

Table 4. Internal and External Forces of Volitional Disorders

A. Predisposition
B. Environment
C. Fortifications
D. Tolerance
E. Physiochemical change
F. Abstinence
G. Hypophoria

Table 5. Etiological Facets of Drug Dependence

1. Inner problems
2. Family
3. Peers
4. Society
5. Culture and values
6. Philosophical problems

Table 6. Components of Volitional Disorders

A. Grandiosity
B. Hypophoria
C. Compulsivity
D. Obsession
E. Lack of control
F. Depression
G. Insecurity
H. Frustration
I. Anxiety

Oftentimes, failure to control impulses and obsessional difficulties result in excessive behavior (eg, drinking bouts and binge eating) that allows one for the moment to overcome personal inadequacies and resort to illusionary powers with the concomitant fulfillment of a fantasy life (grandiosity). Of course if all control is lost then euphoric grandiosity may occur in the fantasies of a complete intoxicated state.

Although some components of the volitional disorders may be described, not all aspects of this extremely complex problem are known. An extensive multifaceted effort (psychological, biochemical, pharmacological, economical, sociological) is required to gain full insight into the nature of these disorders. However, at present millions of individuals suffer at some dysfunctional level from these exaggerated behaviors and often require treatment which must take into consideration the physiological, psychological, and socioeconomic aspects of the problem, but the key to effective therapy is the inner dynamics of the compulsion. In most cases the physiological component of the excessive behavior and the socioeconomic issues can be suitably rectified. The dilemma of course is how can one overcome by sheer willpower the behavior, when the inherent defect is also part of the function. Thus, the compulsions and obsessional difficulties cannot be readily resolved merely by calling upon one's will, determination, and inner strength. The inner dynamics or the psycho-dynamics as I have suggested must be fully understood to successfully treat and resolve the disorder, then and only then might the individual be able to effectively abandon the excessive behavior.

TREATMENT

Let us now examine the various therapeutic modes available for the volitional disorders (Table 7). Certainly the need to alter excessive behavior through behavioral modification (Kokes, 1981) seems obvious. Some success can be obtained with individuals placed in a well-designed multiple component treatment program which involves contingency management, relaxation train-ing, desensitization, covert sensitization, and self-control techniques. It is also important for treatment of this kind that the patient not exhibit signs of chronic psychopathology (ie, psychopath, sociopath). Behavioral therapy, even if not fully effective, is often very useful in the development of behaviors necessary for life management outside the treatment setting.

An extremely interesting theoretical approach to the understanding of volitional disorders is Solomon's opponent-process theory of motivation (Solomon, 1977) in which an initial arousal or response to stimuli is followed by an opposite or opponent process. Unfortunately, the opponent-process system of motivation presents an extremely difficult therapeutic challenge because of the enormous variety of influences that sustain it.

A rather obvious approach to the treatment of excessive behaviors has been suggested by Falk (1981) in which the environment generates and sus-tains the exaggerated behavior. Therefore, an alteration in the environment, the removal of its conditions, or lastly a total change in the environment

Table 7. Treatment

A. Psychodynamics
B. Behavioral modifications
C. Opponent-process motivation
D. Environmental change
E. Self-help (anonymous)
F. Chemotherapy

should be sufficient to provide the necessary therapy to alter the excessive activity. The difficulty with this approach is that the problem is multifaceted and therefore, not easily resolved by altering one condition.

Some success in treating these problems has been achieved by the various anonymous organizations, (A.O.) such as: *alcoholics, obesity,* and *gambling.* These organizations all emphasize the need to rely on a spiritual being or supernatural power for the necessary strength to overcome the exaggerated behavioral activity. In addition to the A.O.s, various drug-free therapeutic communities have also achieved a measure of effectiveness through the combined efforts of both staff and clients in rehabilitating drug abusers.

The major chemotherapeutic approaches as you well know are: opiate agonist (eg, methadone); opiate antagonist (eg, naltrexone); agonist-antagonist (eg, buprenorphine); and the use of major and minor tranquilizers. Some success has been achieved using the drug therapy technique in treating drug abusers, depending somewhat on the criteria used for rehabilitation in a given program.

A valid treatment program for the volitional disorders as indicated previously must be approached from three points of view, (Table 8) namely: (a) physiological, (b) psychological, and (c) socioeconomic (Saltzman, 1980; Wurmster, 1972).

Some addictions like drugs, alcohol, and food, involve all three factors. Others like compulsive sports, compulsive gambling, and overworking seem to be exclusively tied to psychological elements. The psychological factors, however, must transcend and permeate the total program since it is the inner motivational forces that initiate and sustain the disorder and lays the groundwork for the substitution of one behavior for another.

Wurmser (1972) described the interacting facets of the etiology of drug dependence (see Table 5) with a series of six concentric circles: (a) inner problems, (b) family, (c) peer group, (d) society, (e) cultural values, and (f) philosophical problems. The first five relate to psychosocial factors and confirm the impression that psychodynamic insight must be present in the therapy program. An overemphasis on the psychological factors however without altering the physiological or socioeconomic aspects would achieve minimal results with maximum outlays of money.

Table 8. Essential Treatment Components

1. Physiological
2. Psychological
3. Socioeconomic

As with all compulsions, external force, persuasion, threat, humiliation or punishment cannot undo the disorder which has inner dynamics that must be exposed and understood. The addict must be aware of his grandiosity and accept some limitations thereof and commitments to realistic potentials. There is a need to develop techniques for dealing with feelings of powerlessness and helplessness other than through compulsive rituals and illusory feelings of strength and power.

The question again is how does one use determination and will to overcome defects when such defects are due to a disorder of the will; and where the focus and preoccupation on the goal interferes with its attainment? Thus, in the case of compulsion neurotics, they must be healed with the aid of functions that are themselves affected by the disorder. The technique of paradoxical intention, may be useful in this regard since, the destructive behavioral disorder can be overcome by advising and encouraging its persistence. Paradoxically such an emphasis can result in the abandonment of the symptoms. Paradoxical intention is occasionally successful because apparently it removes the focus from overcoming the symptoms, to an exaggeration of them.

Generally, the individual does not enter treatment to terminate the disorder but to get help in making it tolerable or to be relieved of the exhausting effort to maintain it. To abandon compulsive behavior is a matter of finally recognizing one's personal helplessness with the problem. By giving up absolute control over the compulsive behavior reasonable controls may be exerted without grandiose pretensions of invulnerability. The recognition of one's powerlessness cannot be simply verbal, it must go much deeper since, it is the compulsive's verbal capacity that allows circumvention of commitments and maintenance of grandiosity, thereby never really accepting a deficiency.

The achievements of Alcoholics Anonymous illustrate this point even though its success has often been justified by the assumption of a spiritual order rather than psychological readjustments. The process of "surrender" in AA involves the alcoholic's recognition of the compulsive nature of drinking, and the inability to resolve it by will.

Efforts to force or encourage the addict to relinquish the compulsion by willpower, persuasion, moral injunction, etc, will be of no avail. Support for undoing the compulsive behavior must come through the simultaneous recognition of an inner strength and the ability to do so by the combined utilization of physiological, psychological, and socioeconomic resources. Under these conditions an individual may be able to strengthen his capacities for decisive commitment and determined effort to function without the use of chemicals or compulsive rituals. The psychodynamics of excessive behavior, therefore, constitutes the overall umbrella under which all modalities of treatment must operate in order to be successful.

REFERENCES

Falk JL: The environmental generation of excessive behavior. In: SJ Mulé (ed.), *Behavior in Excess: An Examination of the Volitional Disorders.* New York: Free Press, 1981 (in press)

Kokes RF: Behavior therapy in the treatment of behavior in excess. In: SJ Mulé (ed.), *Behavior in Excess: An Examination of the Volitional Disorders.* New York: Free Press, 1981 (in press)

Mulé SJ: Introduction. In: SJ Mulé (ed.), *Behavior in Excess: An Examination of the Volitional Disorders.* New York: Free Press, 1981 (in press)

Saltzman L: Psychodynamics of the addictions. In: SJ Mulé (ed.), *Behavior in Excess: An Examination of the Volitional Disorders.* New York: Free Press, 1981 (in press)

Saltzman L: *Treatment of the Obsessive Personality.* New York: Aronson, 1980

Solomon RL: An opponent-process theory of acquired motivation: IV. The affective dynamics of addiction. In: JD Maser and MEP Seligmans (eds.), *Psychopathology Experimental Models.* WH Freeman Co., pp 66–103, 1977

Wurmster L: Drug abuse-nemesis of psychiatry. *Int J Psychiatry* 10:94–107, 1972

6

Maintenance of Behavior by "Schedules": An Unfamiliar Contribution to Maintenance of Abuses

P.B. DEWS

It has become almost trite to say that drug abuse is the result of many interrelated factors. There is no one single sufficient cause. We are hearing about various factors today. Because there are many contributing factors there are therefore many ways of combating abuse. We should be looking for ways to understand as many of the different contributing factors as possible and learning how to use our knowledge to attack abuse from as many different angles as possible.

The phenomena I am going to talk about today are not the prime factors in initiation of drug abuse, though they may be more important than most people realize in the maintenance of abuse. They are of interest here, because by understanding them we may learn ways to weaken abuse patterns. They also illuminate some hitherto puzzling features of abuses: by seeing a little of what is going on, we can avoid following false trails.

Let me start with an example of a puzzling phenomenon, one that is at the heart of abuse. To any impartial observer the game is not worth the candle. Why does a heroin addict spend so much of his time chasing a fix of heroin when the effects are so trivial and evanescent and the withdrawal syndrome no worse than a dose of flu, indeed much less so for most street "addicts"? Why do alcoholics make themselves dizzy and nauseated and ruin their lives? It has been traditional to assume that with heroin there is a "euphoria" so intense that it overcomes all rational considerations, and that with alcohol there is a desperation to escape which is sufficient to make the distress acceptable. These explanations are ad hoc and there is really no independent evidence adequate to sustain them. What I am going to describe are experiments in animals that show that animals will work, just like addicts, for seemingly inadequate reasons, indeed for consequences that are not merely biologically useless but actually painful.

The only way I can describe the results is by a more or less historical narrative of a series of experiments, mostly performed by my colleagues, W.H. Morse and R.T. Kelleher, over a period of many years. No technical knowledge is necessary to follow the description.

Most of the experiments have been performed in squirrel monkeys which are small primates weighing between 1 and 2 pounds. The animals sit comfortably in so-called restraining chairs, and they have a small lever in front of them, which they can easily press with their hands. Not surprisingly, if they are kept short of food it is relatively easy to get them to press the lever if food is delivered when they do so, even only occasionally. Indeed they will press hundreds of times at rates greater than 1/sec for hours for occasional deliveries of food. Each lever press is called a response. The actual pattern in time of responding depends on the program that determines when food will follow a response; this program is called the schedule, the schedule of reinforcement, and this is the meaning of the term in my title.

An example of a schedule, one that will be important in subsequent discussion, is FI 10 min. It says that a stimulus such as a light comes on, and when it has been on for 600 sec (but only then) a response will produce food. Of course, the subject can respond during the 10 min interval, and indeed that is just what the subject does. When the subject is exposed to this schedule consistently over and over again, several times each day, day after day, a very characteristic pattern of responding develops. At the beginning of the 10 min the subject scarely responds, but when no more than a minute or two have elapsed, responding starts regularly, slowly at first, but increasing in rate smoothly until for the last few minutes of the 600 sec the animal is responding regularly at a rate that may be as high as 1/sec.

This particular pattern of responding is highly characteristic of the schedule. It is by no means just phenomenon of monkeys pressing a lever but has been seen in monkeys pushing a panel or pressing a lever or pulling a bar; dogs pressing a lever or nosing a key or barking; cats pressing a button or meowing; rats pressing a lever, licking or running in a running wheel; mice pressing a lever or breaking a beam of light with their noses or running around a circular track; and pigeons or quail pecking a key. The list is not exhaustive. Nor does the consequence have to be food. Consequences that have been studied include: food, fluid, electric shock, light, dark, warmth, and drug injections; and again the list is not exhaustive. Extensive review is not possible here.

Suffice it to say that for essentially all the pairs of response and consequences that have been studied, in all the species, many aspects of the pattern of responding over time depend on the schedule rather than on the response or the reinforcer. The commonality is amazing. Further, especially with regard to schedules like FI, the pattern of responding in time shows consistency as the parameter value is changed. The pattern that was described for FI 10 min in the monkey is also seen in a pigeon under FI 100,000 sec, which is over 24 hours. For a few hours, the pigeon does not respond, then responding starts, slowly at first then increasing in rate and then occurring steadily over the last several hours of the cycle (Dews, 1965). One feature of schedules that resembles drug abuse is apparent already: a great deal of behavior over long periods of time is controlled by relatively trivial consequences.

We will return to FI but first we must consider some entirely independent lines of experiments that were started almost 45 years ago to try to learn something experimentally about anxiety. The problem of a functional characterization of anxiety was addressed. It was argued that the most important aspect of anxiety may not be the outward manifestation or inward feelings of anxiety but rather the interference with normal behavioral activities.

The following series of experiments in rats were devised. The rats pressed a lever under an FI 4 min schedule of food deliveries. When regular responding was occurring through the 1 hour daily session, a noise was sounded in the middle of the session for 5 min. At the end of the 5-minute noise each day an electric shock was delivered to the feet of the rat through the grid on which it stood. After a number of daily presentations of noise concluded by shock, responding slowed down or ceased during the period of noise, only to resume as soon as the shock had been delivered. The interpretation was that the rat was "anxious" during the noise, anticipating the shock, and the anxiety suppressed normal responding for food during the noise.

Some years later in an entirely different series of experiments, it was shown that a rat would press a lever if that response postponed electric shocks that would otherwide have occurred repeatedly. If, for example, each response postponed the shock for 20 or 30 sec, the rat responded regularly at an average rate much higher than once per 20 or 30 sec, so shocks were received only infrequently. Monkeys performed similarly but so that they even more infrequently received a shock.

What do you suppose would happen if the "anxiety" paradigm is superimposed on responding maintained by shock postponement rather than food delivery? What happened, probably to the surprise of the first workers to make the experiment, was that on the background of postponement respondings the rate increased during the noise preceding inevitable shock rather than decreasing as on the background of responding maintained by food. In subsequent series of experiments it was shown that when no shocks were given except at the end of the noise, so that responding was no longer postponing shock, then respondings ceased except during the noise. During the noise the monkey continued to respond until the delivery of the shock, although, of course, the responding had no influence on the occurrence of the shock or any other programmed event. Thus the animal was responding only when an imminent shock was signaled; so we could say that the shock was maintaining responding.

We now switch to an independent line of experiments. During the 1950s it was shown that the effects of a drug were greatly influenced by the pattern of responding in time on which the drug effect was superimposed. On different rates and patterns, for example, amphetamine could cause either an increase or decrease in rate and the same was true for barbiturates, although different patterns are increased and decreased by the two classes of drugs. Of course, the schedule of reinforcement is the prime determinant of the rate and pattern of responding in time. As described earlier, FI schedules give rise to a smoothly increasing rate of responding through the FI X sec interval, a characteristic pattern consistent across species. FI responding thus provides a whole series of rates in a consistent sequence which can be exposed to the influence of a drug. For many drugs, the effects are different on the different rates. The question was posed: would the drug effects be similar if the drug effect were superimposed on a similar sequence of rates of responding but in reversed order, that is, with the rate at a maximum at the beginning of each cycle and then falling progressively to zero towards the end of cycle?

To try to produce such a pattern, two squirrel monkeys were trained under a VI schedule for food. VI is like FI except that instead of responding during a fixed period of time being concluded by a reinforced response, responding during variable periods of time are concluded by a reinforced response. Typically the periods vary from a few seconds to a few minutes. Such a schedule characteristically maintains a steady, constant rate of responding. On this pattern of sustained responding was superimposed the additional feature that at the end of 10 minutes, for a 1-minute period, every response was followed by a noxious electric shock to the tail. It was anticipated that each cycle might start with responding occurring at full VI rate and then slow down and cease as time approached when a response would produce a shock. In the event, responding in one subject was greatly reduced, especially as the shock became imminent. In the other subject, on the contrary, the frequency of responding during the 10-minute period actually accelerated, so that the subject came to be responding faster and faster as the time approached when a response would produce a shock. The subject came to be responding several times faster just before a response was followed by a shock than at any time under the earlier program when there were no shocks at all.

As soon as the first shock was delivered, however, responding practically ceased until the 1-minute period when every response would be followed by a shock was ended. The pattern of increasing rate of responding up to the time when a shock was delivered brought to mind the previous experiments in which responding that would not otherwise have occurred was maintained by an inevitable shock. Can one go one step further and maintain responding by noxious electric shocks that are a direct consequence of the response, and are thus not inevitable, that is, would not occur if the subject did not press the lever? Can responding be maintained when the only consequence of the response is the occasional delivery of a shock?

Accordingly, in the experiments just described, the delivery of food under the VI schedule was discontinued. The subjects now never received food on pressing the lever; all they could get were electric shocks to the tail at each response in the eleventh minute. The subjects continued to respond through each 10-minute period, however, showing the typical accelerating pattern of FI until a shock was delivered. On delivery of the shock, the monkeys vocalize and thrash around as though the shock were just as noxious and aversive as the same shock is known to be under other circumstances. They then virtually stopped responding for the rest of the 1-minute period when additional shocks would have been delivered, and through a time-out period, only to start again and increase the rate through the next 10-minute period. Thus, we have a subject responding repeatedly, showing a definite FI pattern of rates, when the only consequence of responding is the occasional delivery of a severe, apparently noxious and aversive electric shock under an FI schedule. The shock was highly effective in suppressing responding during the remainder of the 1-minute period of shock availability following the initial shock, so that the shock had not been magically transformed into a different kind of stimulus.

Continued responding when the only consequence of responding is a severe electric shock is not a transient phenomenon. One of the subjects in the original experiments was exposed to some 170 sessions over a period approaching a year, making an average of over 4,000 responses per session or a total of some 700,000 responses, maintained only by occasional shocks. Shock-producing responding was reduced when shock was reduced in intensity and disappeared when shock was removed, only to return when shock was reinstated. In other experiments rhesus monkeys worked steadily, day and night, for 7 days to postpone the delivery of a lesser shock to their tails than the shock the squirrel monkeys were self-administering.

Two points deserve emphasis. One is that the monkeys in the last series of experiments described had never pressed a lever to postpone a shock. It is not, therefore, possible to attribute the maintenance of responding by shocks to spurious shock-postponement responding, as there was no history of postponement. Second, in the later phases of the experiments the monkeys were fully fed, so that responding was not dependent on food deprivation.

Shock-produced patterns of responding have also been generated by yet other different training procedures. Shock-maintained responding has been developed from shock-postponing responding by arranging that the length of time each response postponed the shock became progressively shorter with each succeeding response until it became 0 sec, that is the shock occurred when the last response was made. The original postponement time was then restored and the progressive reduction cycle repeated. Under this procedure, a progressive increase in rate of responding came to occur, ending with the shocked response. Removal of the interim postponing schedule left an FI schedule of shock-presentation to a response. Responding was maintained and the pattern of responding was that characteristic of FI.

The final way of developing shock-maintained responding that will be described involves no independent training. A species may have a high tendency to engage in a particular behavioral activity following an electric shock, for example, attacking and biting other members of the species. If two rats are put together in an enclosure and both given electric shock, the two rats typically rear on their hind legs and bite or attempt to bite one another. If only one subject is present, an inanimate object may be vigorously bitten. A rhesus monkey will bite a drinking spout when an electric shock is delivered to its tail. Such behaviors may occur the first time the shock is delivered. No training is required, and the activity may be similar in all members of a species that are studied and even homologous over a variety of species. Now, squirrel monkeys in laboratories commonly wear collars to which a chain may be attached for ease of handling, for example for taking the monkey from its cage and putting it in a restraining chair. If the chain is left attached to the collar when the monkey is in the chair and a shock is delivered to the tail, the monkey vigorously pulls on the chain. Pulling is seen the first time the shock is delivered, no training is required, and it is a consistent characteristic of squirrel monkeys. If the other end of the chain is attached to a switch activated by pulling the chain then activation of the switch can be made to lead to delivery of a shock, according, for example, to an FI schedule. When electric shocks were delivered the reciprocal processes of shocks producing chain-pulling and chain-pulling producing shocks came into play. Chain-pulling as an elicited response came to be maintained by shock as a consequence.

When shocks were made to occur only on a response, responding was maintained. Significantly, however, the pattern of chain-pulling changed. Initially, each shock delivery was followed by a paroxysm of chain-pulling that subsided into desultory pulling until the next shock started another bout of rapid pulling. As the procedure was continued, the bouts of pulling immediately after the shock became attenuated and pulling increased in frequency through the interval to the next shock just as we would expect for a response controlled by an FI X sec schedule. Thus, in this example, as in the previous ones, it was the schedule that determined the pattern of shock-maintained responding.

Responding maintained by electric shock as the consequence has been shown under FR (a schedule under which the number of responses made determines shock deliveries) as well as FI and the phenomenon has been shown in cats. Because these experiments effectively contradict strongly held prejudices of determinants of behavior, there has been great resistance to accepting them at face value and people have devised absurdly contrived anthropomorphic "explanations" to avoid facing the implications. In retrospect, one can find other instances in the literature of paradoxical effects of noxious stimuli, in which the noxious stimuli increased responding they had been expected to reduce.

We asked at the beginning: as the harm and distress caused by abuses seem so very much greater than the gratification they provide, why do abuses persist? We may not have a final answer, but at least we can now see the phenomenon in a broader context. "Abuse" is not a peculiarity of people and drugs. Perfectly normal experimental animals "abuse" themselves by giving themselves noxious electric shocks as well as by giving themselves drugs. The schedules engender the "abuse" in the animals. Perhaps then schedule type factors play a role in perpetuating drug abuse in humans. The work on schedules has shown that even an unpleasant event, properly scheduled, can maintain a lot of behavior. We don't therefore have to find a predominantly positive effect of a drug to account for it being abused: a bad effect, properly scheduled, could maintain a habit.

Practical consequence follow this line of reasoning. One outstanding feature of schedule controlled behavior is that while it can be very strong and well maintained almost indefinitely—in pharmacological studies we have had monkeys work for hours a day for years; they were doing more or less the same at the end as at the beginning—yet it continues to remain easily modified when the schedule is changed.

Thus, to the extent that schedule factors play a role in human drug abuse, that part, at least, is fully remediable. What sort of a schedule is a heroin addict influenced by? Well, it is a very regular schedule of hustling, making contact to get a fix and then the ritual of taking the drug, pursued so religiously that it may leave little time for other pursuits. How can we interrupt the operation of the schedule? One obvious way is to make the abuser take and keep a job with regular hours. Vaillant in his studies here in New York found in his follow-up of ex denizens of Lexington that by far their best drug-free periods (when they were not institutionalized) was when they had a job that they had to keep (because of a parole requirement that made a condition of freedom the holding of a regular job.)

We know very little about schedule effects in human subjects and it is a very difficult area of research. But research in human subjects will have to be done, before we can really apply laboratory findings to therapy. I believe the benefits, when we learn to apply lab findings to humans, will be great enough to justify the cost and frustrations of doing the work.

ACKNOWLEDGMENT

Original work in this laboratory was supported by U.S. Public Health Service grants MH02094, MH07658, DA00499, and DA02658.

7

Some Endocrine and Immunological Observations In Heroin and Methadone Maintained Opioid Addicts

PAUL CUSHMAN, JR.

The victims of opiate addiction are usually tolerant and physically dependent on opioids during their times of active opiate use. This is the major medical consequence of opiate addiction. In addition, over the years many other medical complications associated with addiction have been reported (Kreek, 1973; White, 1973; Sapira, 1968). Some of these can be related to the life style, habits, and techniques of the opioid user than to the drug effect itself.

We became interested in possible opioid actions on the endocrine system several years ago. This study will review the most important discoveries relating exogenous opioids to the endocrine system in man. The endogenous opioid, enkephalins/endorphins, may play important roles in the endocrine system. This topic is outside the scope of this study. We also studied the immunological consequences of opiate addiction in man, and effects which are much less attributable to the opioids per se.

This report centers on observations made amongst opiate addicts while using street drugs, during methadone maintenance treatment, and after detoxification.

ENDOCRINE OBSERVATIONS

The endocrine system has multiple, interlocking components. It usually has both stimulatory and inhibitory hormones and the balance between the two opposing forces tends to maintain homeostasis. Thus many key body components are kept within an optimal metabolic range. Many of the hormones are regulated by their own blood concentrations or by the products

Table 1. Selected Abnormalities in Opioid Abusers

---

1. Neuroendocrine abnormalities
   a. hypothalamic–pituitary–adrenal axis
   b. hypothalamic–pituitary–gonadal axis
   c. thyroid

2. Immunological disturbances
   a. antibodies related to opiates
      i.   antiheroin antibody–infrequent
   b. antibodies related to style of self-administration of opiates
      i.   immunglobulins
      ii. antibodies *per se*
      iii. cell mediated immune system

---

of their target organ secretion. Both long feedback systems, most extensively worked out for the hypothalamic-pituitary-adrenal (or thyroidal or gonadal) axes, exist as well as short feedback loops where a pituitary hormone may influence its own secretion via a short feedback loop to the hypothalamus.

Study of the opioid effects on hormones must then consider, not only the results of an acute bolus of opioids on a blood concentration of a specific hormone, but also on the dynamics of hormone secretion. Also there are important cellular adjustments that follow long term opioid administration. Tolerance to the agonist effects of opioids occurs with sustained administration (Muslin, 1964; Pradhan, 1977; Eddy, 1965).

Since tolerance develops at non-uniform rates to various opioid agonist effects (Pradhan, 1977) with some (analgesia) rapid, other (antidiarrheal) slowly and other (pupillary) slight if at all, it is important to examine the endocrine effects of exogenous opioids in subjects who have been receiving a fixed daily dose of an opioid (methadone usually) for many months to allow for the complete expression of tolerance.

The chronic opioid users, who are most stable, best documented, most available for study, and most likely to follow an appropriate protocol in which specified baseline conditions are desired, are the methadone maintenance recipients.

HYPOTHALAMIC-PITUITARY-ADRENAL AXIS

Several animal and human studies raise questions about the effects of acute opioids on the HPA axis (Kokka, 1974; George, 1976; Fishman, 1977; Van Vugt, 1980). Some data suggest the opioids stimulate ACTH-cortisol release, and others imply that there may be lesser ACTH-cortisol secretion after opioids than would be expected without them (Briggs, 1955; Reier, 1973; McDonald, 1959). Because of its importance, careful study of the HPA axis in relation to opioids is warranted.

Table 2. Hypothalamic–Pituitary–Adrenal Axis

1. Low Opioid Tolerance–ie, "street level"
   a. unstimulated plasma cortisol . . . . normal
   b. plasma cortisol responses to hypoglycemia (stress). . . . normal
   c. unstimulated plasma ACTH . . . . low ←→ normal (Ho et al)
   d. urine corticosteroid responses to metyrapone. . . . . . . low (Kreek)

2. High Opioid Tolerance–ie, (40–100 mg/day methadone)
   a. unstimulated plasma cortisol . . . . normal
   b. plasma cortisol responses to hypoglycemia, ACTH. . . . normal
   c. urine corticosteroid responses to metyrapone. . . . . . . normal
   d. cortisol secretion rate . . . . normal (Hellman et al)

Most data are reassuring, indicating that the HPA axis was normal or near normal in the non-tolerant subjects given acute opioids. The low-tolerance (street drug using) opiate addict (Table 2), usually had normal plasma cortisol and near normal levels ACTH when resting (unstimulated) conditions (Ho, 1977; Cushman, 1970). HPA dynamics revealed normal responses to exogenous ACTH (Eisenman, 1961); insulin hypoglycemia, which measures the HPA axis response to stress, is normal (Cushman, 1970). Metyrapone, an adrenal inhibitor of 11b hydroxylase which reduces plasma cortisol and invokes ACTH secretion via the feedback route, produced initially a low response in urinary 17 ketogenic steroids in a small number of patients. Later their responses were normal (Cushman, 1970).

The tolerant methadone recipients, tolerant to 40–100 mg of oral methadone daily, showed normal plasma cortisol levels for the most part, normal increases in HPA axis after metyrapone and insulin hypoglycemia (Cushman, 1981) and normal cortisol secretion rates (Hellman, 1975).

HYPOTHALAMIC-PITUITARY GONADAL AXIS

In contrast to the HPA axis, there are abundant data showing opioid related adverse effects on the HPG axis. Clinical reports of infertility, fluctuating libido, erectile problems, delayed orgasm, disordered menstruation are common (Cushman, 1972; Wieland, 1970). Seventy to ninety percent of females, who reported normal menses prior to opiate addiction, had menstrual disturbances during addiction. Since most were normal after detoxification (Santen, 1975; Gaulden, 1964; Stoffer, 1968), the data strongly suggest that something associated with addiction was causative of their menstrual abnormalities.

Hormone studies have been extensively performed on males. Resting (unstimulated) blood levels of FSH, LH, and Prolactin are listed in Table 3. Low LH and to a much lesser extent low FSH levels were frequent amongst

Table 3. Hypothalamic–Pituitary–Gonadal Axis

1. Low Opiate Tolerant Persons–"street level"	
a. resting or unstimulated FSH . . . . ↓	
b. resting or unstimulated LH . . . . ↓	
c. prolactin* . . . . ↑ variable	
d. plasma testosterone levels . . . . ↓	
e. stimulated FSH/LH . . . . ↓ (Brambilla)	
2. Opiate Tolerant Persons (40–100 mg/day methadone)	
a. unstimulated FSH . . . . N/↓ occasionally (Azizi)	
b. unstimulated LH . . . . N/↓ occasionally	
c. stimulated LF, FSH (IV LRH) . . . . Normal (Dent)	
d. prolactin . . . . ↑/N (Kreek, Dent)	
e. unstimulated . . . . often ↑ after next opioid dose	
f. serum testosterone T . . . . low ←→ normal	
g. serum estradiol E2 . . . . normal ←→ low (Azizi)	

Studies done in males unless *, whereupon studies done in both genders.

low tolerance, street drug opiate addicts (Azizi, 1973; Brambilla, 1979).
Prolactin levels were variable. With high tolerance as to methadone, most
patients had normal LH, FSH, and prolactin levels (Cushman, 1974). Stimulation of LH/FSH levels with exogenous LRH were subnormal in a group of
Italian street addicts (Brambilla, 1979), but normal amongst a group of
methadone maintained patients (Dent, 1975).

Plasma testosterone levels amongst opioid addicts ranged widely, with
many individual values below the range of normal (Mendelson, 1975;
Cushman, 1973; Cicero, 1975). Amongst methadone-maintained patients the
plasma testosterone (T) levels tended to be lower in those who had high
daily methadone dose; an inverse relationship between plasma T and daily
methadone was found. In an inpatient controlled setting, acute opioids
lowered plasma LH and T, and their discontinuation was accompanied by a
rapid return of plasma T to normal (Mendelson, 1975).

PRL rises in the normal subject after an acute bolus of opioids
(Fishman, 1977; Cushman, 1974). This phenomenon is well studied with
animals. Considerable evidence imply that it may involve dopamine at the
hypothalamic level. Opioid tolerant persons, usually, but not invariably,
retain their capacity to augment their PRL level after additional opioid doses
(Cicero, 1975). Most male opioid users had normal estradiol levels (Azizi,
1973) and secretion rates (Cushman, 1974).

Amongst females, hormone studies have been relatively sparse. In
detailed studies of a few females with histories of oligo-amenorrhea by
Santen (1975), there was less evidence of hypothalamic inhibition of LH
surges and anovulation. To what extent these findings apply to the other
female addicts is unclear.

Table 4. Thyroid Function Tests in Opiate Addicts

1. Low Tolerance–"street" addict
   a. Thyroxine (T4) . . . . ↑ normal
   b. Tri-iodothyronine (T3) resin uptake . . . . ↓ normal
   c. Thyroxine binding globulin capacity . . . . ↑
   d. TSH . . . . normal

2. High Tolerance–methadone patients (20–100 mg/gd)
   a. T4 . . . . usually N, occasionally ↑
   b. T3 resin . . . . usually N, occasionally ↓
   c. TSH . . . . normal

THYROID

The thyroid-TSH axis appears to function normally in both low and high levels of opioid tolerance. The major finding was in the laboratory measurements of thyroid function. Common amongst street addicts was a high serum thyroxine (T4), and reduced T3 resin uptakes (Webster, 1973; Azizi, 1974). Their euthyroid status was attested to by their normal TSH and free T4 levels. The difficulty seemed to be related to augmentation of the binding capacity of Thyroxine Binding Globulin (TBG). This abnormality, which may relate to liver disease or to relatively low androgenicity appeared to become less common after methadone maintainence treatment (Webster, 1973; Table 4).

IMMUNOLOGICAL

Application of immunological tools to human opioid addicts disclosed a variety of abnormalities.

Heroin itself is poorly antigenic (Azizi, 1974); hence very little of the humoral changes could be accounted for by the development of anti-heroin antibodies. On the other hand, circulating immune complexes were common (Smith, 1975; Bayer, 1976; Table 5). Yet very little immune complex disease manifestations were observed. Occasionally, a heroin addict will show the nephrotic syndrome with immune bodies identified in the glomeruli, but very few patients show arthritis, purpura, vasculities, etc. Studies of cell mediated immunity are far from complete and have produced conflicting results. Blast transformation using phytohemagglutinnin may or may not be altered in heroin addiction (Ortona, 1979). Our studies of E rosette (early type) amongst opioid addicts found a mixed bag, which defied interpretation (Brown, 1974); others (Cushman, 1973) found a depression. There did not

Table 5. Immune Measurements in Opioid Addicts

---

1. Immune Complexes
   a. ↑ 41–54.8% (Bayer-Ortura)

2. Cell Mediated Immunity
   a. Phytohemagglutinin stimulated–N ⟷ low
   b. Early (E) Rosettes–variable ↑ N ↓

3. Antibody Classes
   a. IgM–↑ 40–80%
   b. IgG–↑ 20–50%
   c. IgA–normal
   d. IgD–normal

4. Antibodies
   a. CMV–↑ in 11% (Grieco)
   b. Latex fixation–↑ in 25%
   c. Biological false + test for syphilis (Reagin)–↑ in 25%

---

seem to be impairment of delayed tuberculin type skin test hypersensitivity in the addict.

On the other hand, there are numerous abnormalities in the other arm of the immune system. Antibody classes, especially IgM and to a lesser extent IgG, were often abnormally high amongst individual addicts, as well as being strikingly high amongst populations of addicts compared to controls. No changes in IgA or IgD were found (Cushman, 1973; Grieco, 1973).

With methadone treatment, perhaps related to sharp reduction in the rates of parenteral drug use, serial IgM levels tended to return to normal in a prospective study. Other clinical antibody measurements are high amongst opioid addicts (Millian, 1971). Rheumatoid factors, and the biological false positive tests for syphilis (BFP) were only a few of the many more common antibody titers which were found to be inappropriately high (or abnormally present) amongst opioid addicts. Other antibody levels, as anti CMV or anti hepatitis B, are probably high as a consequence of infection. Ratio of BFP fell with methadone treatment, time, and possibly amelioration of liver disease (Table 6; Cushman, 1974).

Since heroin is poorly antigenic, since the increased serum IgM was primarily seen amongst parenteral drug users rather than those using intranasal route for drug administration, and since many infections with yeasts, bacteria, fungi, protozoa, and viruses have been observed amongst opioid addicts, it may be presumed that the humoral immunological changes were caused by diluents, filter, infections, or contaminants acquired along with the opioid rather than caused by the opioid per se.

Table 6. Methadone Treatment and Serological Tests for Syphilis
in Opiate Addicts

	N	Positive	With Syphilis	False +*
Entrants into Methadone maintenance	69	36%	13%	23%
Same Methadone recipients after 23 ± 7 months of ℞	69	12%	6%	6%
Control opiate addicts	94	23%	2%	21%
Controls (normals)	875	1%	–	0.7%

*VDRL positive, fluorescent treponemal antibody negative.

IN CONCLUSION

The opioid user may have a variety of endocrine disturbances, most importantly involving the hypothalamic-pituitary-gonadal axis. No clinically significant problems with the ACTH-cortisol were found. Laboratory testing of thyroid function showed high TGB capacities, but no abnormality in thyroid function.

The cell mediated immune system, inadequately studied, may be near normal since the present adverse data are not convincing. The humoral immune system appears vigorous, if not over stimulated, responding to a variety of antigens. Methadone treatment generally was accompanied by fewer abnormalities, with the exception of testosterone, where an inverse relationship with dose of methadone and plasma testosterone was observed. Methadone treatment was usually accompanied by fewer endocrine and humoral abnormalities after compared to before treatment.

REFERENCES

Azizi F, Vagenakis AG, Longcope C, et al: Decreased serum testosterone levels in male heroin addicts. *Steroids* 22:467–472, 1973

Azizi F, Vagenakis AG and Portnay GI: Thyroxine transport and metabolism in methadone and heroin addicts. *Ann Intern Med* 80:194–199, 1974

Bayer AS, Theofilopoulos R and Eisenberg R: Circulating immunecomplexes in infective endocarditis. *N Engl J Med* 295:1500–1502, 1976

Brambilla F, Resele L, DeMaio D, et al: Gonadotropin response to synthetic hormone (GnRH) in heroin addicts. *Am J Psychiatry* 163:314–316, 1979

Briggs F and Munson P: Studies on the mechanism of stimulation of ACTH secretion with the aid of morphine as a blocking agent. *Endocrinology* 57:205–209, 1955

Brown SM, Stimmel B and Taub RN: Immunological dysfunction in heroin addicts. *Arch Intern Med* 134:1001–1004, 1974

Cicero TJ, Bell RD, Wiest WG, et al: Function of the male sex organs in heroin and methadone users. *New Engl J Med* 292:882–887, 1975

Cushman P: Narcotic and hormones. *Advances in Substance* 1:000–000, 1981

Cushman P: Plasma testosterone in narcotic addiction. *Amer J Med* 55:452–457, 1973

Cushman P: Sexual behavior in heroin addiction and methadone maintenance. *New York State J Med* 72:1721–1923, 1972

Cushman P, Bordier B and Hilton JG: Hypothalamic-pituitary-adrenal axis in methadone treated heroin addicts. *J Clin Endocrinol Metab* 30:607–612, 1970

Cushman P and Grieco MH: Hyperimmunolglobulinemia with narcotic addiction. *Am J Med* 54:320–325, 1973

Cushman P, Gupta S and Grieco MH: Immunological studies in methadone maintained patients. *Int J Addict* 12:241–244, 1977

Cushman P and Kreek MJ: Methadone maintained patients. *New York State J Med* 74:1970–1970, 1974

Cushman P and Kreek MJ: Some endocrinologic observations in narcotic addicts. In: R Zimmermann and R George (eds.), *Narcotics and the Hypothalamus*. New York: Raven Press, pp 161–173, 1974

Cushman P and Sherman CA: Biologic false positive reactions in serological tests for syphilis in narcotic addiction. *Am J Clin Path* 61:346–351, 1974

Dent R and Tolis G: Hypothalamic-pituitary target organ axis in patients on methadone maintenance. *Endocrine Society Annual Meeting Proceedings*, p 217, 1975

Eddy N, et al: Drug dependence: Its significance and characteristics. *Bull World Health Organ* 32:721–733, 1965

Eisenman AJ, Fraser HF and Brooks JW: Urinary excretion and plasma levels of 17 hydroxycorticosteroids during a cycle of addiction to morphine. *J Pharm Exp Ther* 132:131–134, 1961

Fishman J: The opiates and the endocrine system. In: J Fishman (ed.), *Bases of Addiction*. Dahlem Konferenzen, pp 257–280, 1977

Gaulden EC, Littlefield DC and Putoff OE: Menstrual abnormalities associated with heroin addiction. *Am J Obstet Gynecol* 90:155–159, 1964

George JM, Reier CE and Lanse RA: Morphine anesthesia blocks cortisol and growth hormone response to surgical stress in humans. *J Clin Endocrinol Metab* 38:736–743, 1976

Grieco MH and Chuang CY: Hypermacroglobulinemia associated with heroin use in adolescents. *J Allergy Clin Immunol* 51:152–156, 1973

Hellman L, Fukushima DK and Roffwarg H: Changes in estradiol and cortisol production rates in men under the influence of narcotics. *J Clin Endocrinol Metab* 41:1014–1019, 1975

Ho EEK, Ern HL, Fung KP, et al: Comparison of plasma hormone levels between heroin addicts and normal subjects. *Clinica Chemica Acta* 75:415–419, 1977

Kokka N and George R: Effects of narcotic analgesics, anesthetics and hypothalamic lesions on growth hormone and ACTH secretion in rats. In: E Zimmerman and R George (eds.), *Narcotics and the Hypothalamus*. New York: Raven Press, pp 137–159, 1974

Kreek MJ: Medical safety and side effects of methadone in tolerant individuals. *JAMA* 223:665–689, 1973

McDonald RK, Evans FT, Weise YK, et al: Effect of morphine and nalorphine on plasma hydrocortisone levels in man. *J Pharmacol Exp Ther* 125:241–247, 1959

Mendelson JH, Meyer RE, Ellingboe J, et al: Effects of heroin and methadone on plasma cortisol and testosterone. *J Pharmacol Exp Ther* 195:296–302, 1975

Millian SJ and Cherbin CE: Serologic investigations in narcotic addicts. *Am J Clin Path* 56:693–698, 1971

Muslin BE, Grell R and Cochin J: Studies on tolerance: The role of the interval between doses on the development of tolerance to morphine. *J Pharm Exp Therap* 145:1–13, 1964

Ortona L, Laghi V and Gauda R: Immune function in heroin addict. *New Engl J Med* 300:45–47, 1979

Pradhan SN and Dutta SN: *Narcotic Analgesics in Drug Abuse: Clinical and Basic Aspects.* SN Pradhan and SN Dutta (eds.). St. Louis: CV Mosby Co, p 67, 1977

Reier CE, George LM and Kliman JW: Cortisol and growth hormone response to surgical stress during morphine analgesia. *Anesthesia Analgesia* 52:1003–1006, 1973

Santen RJ, Sofsky J, Bilic N, et al: Mechanism of action of narcotics in the production of menstrual dysfunction in women. *Fertil Steril* 26:538–548, 1975

Sapira JD: The narcotic addicts as a medical patients. *Am J Med* 45:555–588, 1968

Smith WR, Wells ID and Glauser FL: Immunological studies in heroin lung. *Chest* 68:651–655, 1975

Stoffer SS: A gynecological study of drug addicts. *Am J Obstet Gynecol* 101:799–804, 1968

Van Vugt DF and Meites J: Influence of exogenous opiates on anterior pituitary function *Fed Proc* 39:2533–2538, 1980

Webster JB, Coupal JJ and Cushman P: Increased thyroxine levels in euthyroid narcotic addicts. *J Clin Endocrinol Metab* 37:928–934, 1973

White AG: Medical disorders in drug addicts. *J Am Med Assn* 223:1469–1471, 1973

Wieland WE and Younger M: Sexual effects and side effects of heroin and methadone. Proceedings Third National Conference on Methadone Treatment. Washington, DC, 1970

8

Multiple Opiate Receptors

R. SUZANNE ZUKIN
STEPHEN R. ZUKIN

HETEROGENEITY OF OPIATE SUBJECTIVE BEHAVIORAL EFFECTS

Opiates, a large class of "morphine-like" drugs, exert a large range of pharmacological effects, in addition to analgesia. The heterogeneity of effects among opiates has been well known for many years. Most notable in this regard are the properties of the mixed agonist-antagonist opiates of the benzomorphan series. These compounds have been of special interest because of the desirability of developing a drug having morphine-like analgesic effects but lacking addictive potential. Cyclazocine, SKF-10,047 (N-allylnor-cyclazocine), and related drugs of the benzomorphan group differ from classical opiates in displaying psychotomimetic effects in humans and unique behavioral effects in animals (Haertzen, 1970; Holtzman, 1979). The syndromes associated with many of the benzomorphans depend dramatically on the species and vary qualitatively with the dose administered. At low doses many of these drugs produce effective analgesia in humans (Lasagna, 1954; Keats, 1964). In addition, they may clinically antagonize the analgesic and respiratory-depressant effects of classical opiates (Harris, 1964), precipitate a withdrawal syndrome in morphine-addicted patients, and prevent development of addiction to morphine (Martin, 1965). At the same time, these opiates may produce physical dependence when administered alone and a characteristic withdrawal syndrome differing from that of morphine upon drug cessation (Martin, 1965). At higher doses such benzomorphans produce a combination of sedation, "drunkenness," and psychosis differing from any morphine effect (Harris, 1964; Martin, 1967). The psychotomimetic effects include depersonalization, dysphoria, suspiciousness, and hallucinations (Haertzen, 1970).

77

In animal behavioral studies these drugs also produce both classical opiate (Killam, 1976; Steinert, 1973) and unique effects. The latter include disruption of learned avoidance performances (Wray, 1972) and locomotor stimulation not reversed by naloxone (Holtzman, 1973), constriction of pupils, decreases in flexor reflex and skin twitch, sedation, ("K" effects) and/or canine delirium, tachycardia and tachypnea ("σ" effects) (Gilbert, 1976; Martin, 1976). On the basis of its properties in dogs, cyclazocine was proposed to be a μ antagonist, K agonist, and σ agonist (Martin, 1976); SKF-10,047 was proposed to be a more selective μ antagonist and σ agonist with relatively few K properties (Gilbert, 1976).

Certain of the effects of SKF or cyclazocine in animals cannot be reversed by the pure opiate antagonists naloxone or naltrexone (Holtzman, 1969; Teal, 1980; Rosencrans, 1978). Other effects of these can be so reversed, but only at significantly higher antagonist concentrations that are required to reverse morphine actions (Schaefer, 1978; Jasinski, 1968; Lord, 1977). Thus, in humans and in animals the mixed agonist-antagonist opiates produce a combination of morphine-like effects, anti-morphine effects, and unique sedative and psychotomimetic effects.

OPIATE RECEPTOR SUBCLASSES

The wide diversity of behavioral effects exhibited by these opiate analgesics raises the question as to whether these could be mediated by a single class of receptor sites. Heterogeneous opiate receptor populations were postulated by Martin and coworkers (1976) on the basis of neurophysiological and behavioral evidence. Striking differences in pharmacological responses to different types of narcotic analgesics and their inabilities to substitute for one another in the suppression of withdrawal symptoms in addicted animals provided evidence for at least three receptor types in the dog CNS. These were termed (1) μ receptors with which morphine-like drugs preferentially interact; (2) K receptors with which some benzomorphans such as keto-cyclazocine interact; and (3) σ receptors, for which the prototypic ligand is N-allylnorcyclazocine (SKF-10,047). Effects associated with μ receptors included meiosis, bradycardia, hypothermia, analgesia and indifference. Effects characteristic of the K receptor included pupillary constriction, decreased flexor reflexes and sedation. The σ syndrome involved mydriasis, tachycardia, and mania or "canine delirium," which Martin proposed to be the equivalent of psychotomimetic effects in man.

More recently the evidence for distinct β-endorphin, enkephalin, and possible dynorphin-mediated neuronal systems has lent support to the concept of multiple opiate receptors. In pharmacological and biochemical investigations, Kosterlitz and his co-workers (Lord, 1977) provided evidence for yet a fourth opiate receptor type. The δ receptor was postulated to be the site at which the shorter enkephalin peptides preferentially interact. The depression of electrically-induced contractions in the guinea pig ileum and mouse vas deferens and the inhibition of radiolabelled opiate binding in brain were used as assays. The guinea pig ileum was shown to contain mainly μ receptors, whereas the mouse vas deferens contained a mixture of μ and the putative δ receptor, with which the shorter enkephalin peptides preferentially interact. Thus, in the ileum, enkephalins are equal or slightly less potent than morphine whereas in the vas deferens, stable synthetic enkephalins are about 200 times more potent than is morphine. In addition, the guinea pig ileum would appear, on the basis of pharmacological evidence, to have many more K receptors than does the mouse vas deferens. Guinea pig brain appeared to parallel the mouse vas deferens most nearly in its receptor subclass distribution. By contrast, many neutoblastoma cell lines have been shown to bear only enkephalin or δ receptors (Chang, 1978).

How mutually exclusive are the opiate receptor subtypes? On the basis of clinical and animal behavioral studies alone it is not possible to determine whether putative σ ligands, for example, exert their effects through a unique population of "σ" receptors alone or whether they cross-react with μ and σ receptors. In addition, such studies cannot determine whether there are distinct μ, K, and σ receptors, or whether the diverse effects of these opiates are mediated by binding in different manners to the same receptor.

Of particular interest is the finding that in pharmacological assays, β-endorphin, unlike the shorter opioid peptides, interacts equally well with both μ and δ receptors. This result suggests that met-enkephalin may be designed for a more specialized function than β-endorphin. Recently, Snyder (1980) has suggested that met-enkephalin may be the endogenous ligand specifically targeted for mu receptors, whereas leuenkephalin is the endogenous delta ligand. We have prepared a radioiodinated sulfoxide-carbinol derivative of met^5-enkephalin, FK 33-824 (Roemer, 1977), and have shown by competitive displacement analyses that this shorter opioid peptide also interacts equally well with the putative μ and δ receptors (Kream, 1979). On the basis of studies with enkephalin fragments, Chang and Cuatrecasas (1979) have suggested that it may be the hydrophobic group of the phenylalanine residue of enkephalin which is responsible for recognition by δ receptors.

Among the narcotic opiates N-cyclopropylmethylnoretorphine and some mixed agonist-antagonist opiates appear to be equipotent in competing with μ and δ ligands and thus appear to interact equally well with both receptor types (Chang, 1979).

BIOCHEMICAL EVIDENCE FOR MU AND DELTA RECEPTORS

Substantiation for heterogenous opiate receptors comes from a variety of pharmacological and biochemical approaches. Differences in pharmacological profiles of opiates and opioid peptides provide the first *in vitro* evidence for the existence of distinct opiate receptor subtypes (Lord, 1977; Waterfield, 1977; Simantov, 1978; Lord, 1976; Kosterlitz, 1980). In particular, comparison of the results of binding studies in the brain with those of bioassays in preparations innervated by cholinergic or adrenergic nerves suggested that opiate receptor populations in both the central and peripheral systems are heterogeneous (Lord, 1977; Lord, 1976). Opiate narcotic agonists and antagonists were found to be more potent inhibitors of the binding of labelled opiates than of labelled enkephalins, whereas the reverse was found to be true of enkephalins and their analogs. Conclusions were based on the observation that the rank order of potency was different in different assay systems.

More recently, studies involving the competition of ligands for radio-labelled opiate binding sites in specific brain regions (Chang, 1979; Simantov, 1978; Leslie, 1980) have provided further biochemical evidence for mu and delta receptors, and indicate that these have somewhat different distributions throughout the brain. Thus the thalamus and hypothalamus were shown to be relatively enriched in mu receptors. In contrast, the frontal cortex and striatum appeared to have equivalent densities of these receptor types. These results have been confirmed by light microscopy autoradiography studies (Goodman, 1980) involving ^{125}I-[D-Ala^a, MePhe^4, Met(0)^5-ol] enkephalin as a μ ligand and ^{125}I-[D-Ala^2, D-Leu^5] enkephalin as the δ probe.

A direct and elegant approach has been that of cross-protection studies. Thus, it is expected that for the protection of a specific opiate receptor class against inactivation by alkylating agents, alkaloid opiates would protect alkaloid binding sites more effectively than would the enkephalins. Conversely, the enkephalin binding sites would be expected to be more effectively protected by enkephalins than by alkaloids. Using just such an approach, Robson and Kosterlitz (1979) showed that dihydromorphine (DHM) protects against inactivation of [^{3}H] DHM binding sites by phenoxybenzamine more effectively than does D-Ala^2, D-Leu^5-enkephalin. Similarly, DADLE protects [^{3}H] DADLE sites more effectively than does DHM. At the same time Simon and co-workers (Smith, 1980) showed that naltrexone and morphine are 20 and 8 times, respectively, more effective in protecting the binding of [^{3}H] naltrexone than of [^{3}H] enkephalin against inactivation by N-ethylmaleimide. DADLE and D-Ala^2, Met^5-enkephalinamide (DALA), however, were more effective (7 and 30 times, respectively) for the protection of [^{3}H] DADLE binding. Together these studies have provided considerable substantiation for mu and delta receptors.

What is the molecular basis of these receptor differences? Possible molecular models include: (1) that μ, δ, and other opiate receptors may be distinct polypeptide chains, the 3-dimensional structures of which are related but not identical; or (2) that these subclasses are the same polypeptide species in different lipid or membrane environments, in different conformational or aggregation states, or in the presence or absence of small effector-regulator molecules. Solubilization of the receptor species and its eventual purification and characterization should provide the size, subunit composition, and structural information to distinguish among these and other possibilities.

Although opiate receptor subclasses have been shown to differ with respect to ligand specificity, their interrelationships at the cellular level and possible functional distinctions have not been determined. Preliminary studies by ourselves (Zukin, 1980) and by others (Pert, 1980) suggest that μ receptor binding may be significantly more sensitive to negative regulation by guanyl nucleotides than δ receptor binding. Thus, μ receptors could be functionally coupled to adenyl cyclase and δ receptors not. Other approaches which would provide clarification of this issue include localization of opiate receptor subtypes to pre- or postsynaptic membranes, in specific brain regions, and in peripheral tissue.

ARE THERE REALLY KAPPA AND SIGMA RECEPTORS?

Whereas a wide body of tantalizing data has provided evidence for the existence of distinct mu and delta receptors, attempts to establish the presence of kappa and sigma receptors have been more difficult. Thus, the first *in vitro* receptor binding studies involving [^{3}H] ethylketocyclazocine (EKC, putative mu and kappa ligand) (Hiller, 1979; Pasternak, 1980; Chang, 1980; Kosterlitz, 1980) concluded that there were no distinct kappa receptors in brain. These investigations involved competitive displacement analyses and regional distribution studies of the [^{3}H] EKC high affinity binding component only. These parameters were then compared with those previously reported for radiolabelled-μ ligands. Other studies, notably those of Kosterlitz and Paterson (1980) and of Romer et al (1980), did lend support to the concept of kappa sites. The former showed in cross protection studies that EKC was far more effective than was morphine in preventing the inactivation of [^{3}H] EKC binding sites by phenoxybenzamine. One possible explanation for these differing conclusions was that the Kosterlitz group worked with guinea pig brain, which they showed to have four times the density of kappa receptors than does rat brain. Romer and his co-workers (1980) studied the pharmacology and binding properties of bremazocine, a drug which they proposed to be a highly selective K agonist. *In vivo,* bremazocine produced both potent and analgesia, and the K syndrome previously described by Martin for keto-cyclazocine. No cross-tolerance to morphine was observed. In the guinea pig ileum and mouse vas deferens assays, bremazocine inhibition of electrically-induced contractions was reversible by MR 2266 but not by naloxone. Binding of [^{3}H] bremazocine occurred to a single class of sites with a high affinity (K_D = 0.55nM). In competition displacement analyses, MR 2266 and WIN 44,441-3 were shown to be much more potent than was morphine. Together these findings provide strong evidence that bremazocine interacts with non-μ opiate receptors, most likely K receptors.

Important evidence for K and σ receptors has also been provided in two recent behavioral studies. Harris (1980) using the scheduled-controlled behavior paradigm and Holtzman (1980) using the drug-discriminative stimulus assay have provided convincing evidence that μ, K, and σ drugs each interact with distinct receptors.

Our approach has been to study the binding sites of [^{3}H] cyclazocine (putative μ, K, and σ ligand), [^{3}H] EKC, and [^{3}H] SKF-10,047 (putative mu and sigma ligand) by a combination of Scatchard, competitive displacement, and kinetic analyses (Zukin, 1981). In the first set of studies, we measured specific [^{3}H] cyclazocine binding, defined as total binding minus binding in the presence of 1 μM non-radioactive cyclazocine, as a function of [^{3}H] cyclazocine concentration. Specific binding was found to constitute approximately 92 percent of total binding at 1.0 nM [^{3}H] ligand and 67 percent of total binding at 100 nM [^{3}H] ligand. Binding data obtained using a centrifugation assay were shown to vary less than ± 5 percent from that obtained using the rapid filtration assay. Scatchard analyses revealed the interaction of [^{3}H] cyclazocine with three distinct binding sites characterized by affinities of 0.2 nM, 10 nM and 70 nM (50 mM Tris-HCl buffer, pH 7.4 at 4°C). In contrast, many radiolabelled classical opiates and opioid peptides exhibit biphasic binding, but do not exhibit binding to such a low affinity site.

The apparent K_D of 0.2 nM for the high affinity cyclazocine site agreed closely with that reported for displacement by cyclazocine of [^{3}H] naloxone binding to the opiate receptor. Addition of 15 nM naloxone to the incubation mixture resulted in elimination of [^{3}H] cyclazocine binding to the tight sites with relatively little change in binding to the weak sites. When a series of opiates were tested for their abilities to displace specifically bound [^{3}H] cyclazocine (1 nM), their rank order agreed with that for their displacement of [^{3}H] naloxone. Together these findings indicated that the high affinity cyclazocine binding was occurring to the classical opiate receptor.

The only drugs other than cyclazocine-like opiates which proved active at displacing [^{3}H] cyclazocine from the site of lowest affinit were PCP-like drugs. The relative potencies of a series of PCP analogs in displacement of

[³H] cyclazocine (60 nM) in the presence of naloxone (60 nM) were similar to those for their abilities to displace [³H] PCP from its binding sites (Zukin, 1979; Zukin, 1981). The binding affinity of 70 nM observed for [³H] cyclazocine binding to the weak sites was consistent with the IC_{50} of 200 nM observed for displacement of [³H] PCP by cyclazocine. The total number of weak cyclazocine binding sites (820 fmol/mg protein) was similar to that of specific PCP sites (1100 fmol/mg protein) measured under the same conditions using polylysine-soaked filters. Addition of PCP (10 μM) to the incubation mixture resulted in the disappearance of [³H] cyclazocine binding to the weak (70 nM) sites. Together, these findings suggested that the "low affinity" [³H] cyclazocine binding was occurring to the [³H] PCP binding site.

The high and low affinity [³H] cyclazocine sites exhibited differential sensitivities to sodium and also to the selective sulfhydryl reagent N-ethyl-maleimide. In addition, all three sites exhibited greater than 50 percent loss of specific binding following incubation with trypsin (5 μg/ml) for 15 min at room temperature, and greater than 80 percent loss of specific binding following incubation at 60°C for 15 min in the absence of added reagents. Together, these findings indicated that all three sites have a proteinlike component.

In summary, competition analyses involving rank order determinations for a series of opiates and other drugs have indicated that the cyclazocine binding sites represent, in order of decreasing affinity: (1) the classical opiate receptor (the putative "μ" receptor); (2) a second as yet uncharacterized opiate binding site; and (3) the specific [³H] phencyclidine binding site.

In a second set of studies, we have studied the binding of [³H] EKC and [³H] SKF-10,047 to rat brain homogenates in order to provide further evidence for kappa and sigma receptors, and to attempt to understand the diverse actions of these drugs (Zukin, 1981). Scatchard analyses utilizing various competing drugs revealed the apparent interaction of [³H] EKC with two binding sites with affinities of 0.3 nM (B_{max} = 75 fmol/mg) and 22 nM (B_{max} = 60 fmol/mg). DHM or DADLE (20 nM) reduced [³H] EKC binding to high-affinity sites by approximately 50 percent but had no significant effect on binding to low-affinity sites. DHM (100 nM) plus DADLE (20 nM) reduced [³H] EKC binding to high-affinity sites by more than 90 percent while not affecting binding to weak sites. A series of opiates displaced binding of [³H] EKC from high-affinity sites in rank order bremazocine > EKC > cyclazocine > DHM > DADLE while not affecting low-affinity [³H] EKC binding. Phencyclidine (PCP) selectively displaced [³H] EKC binding from low-affinity sites. The high- and low-affinity [³H] EKC sites exhibited differential sensitivities to sodium. For [³H] SKF-10,047 Scatchard analyses again revealed two distinct binding sites characterized by affinities of 4 nM (B_{max} = 160 fmol/mg) and 65 nM (B_{max} = 800 fmol/mg).

Normorphine (100 nM) markedly reduced binding of [^{3}H] SKF-10,047 to only the high-affinity sites. Rank orders for opiate displacement of 4 nM [^{3}H] SKF-10,047 were bremazocine = cyclazocine = levorphanol > SKF-10,047 > DADLE > morphine > pentazocine. PCP selectively decreased low-affinity SKF-10,047 binding. These data provide biochemical evidence for interaction of EKC and SKF-10,047 with the σ receptor (which we have previously identified with the PCP receptor) and the μ receptor. The high-affinity EKC binding may represent a combination of μ and K receptor populations.

ARE THE SIGMA RECEPTOR AND [^{3}H] PCP BINDING SITE ONE AND THE SAME?

Another analgesic and anesthetic drug with prominent psychotomimetic side effects is phencyclidine (PCP, or "angel dust"). Early trials in humans showed PCP to produce excellent anesthesia and analgesia (Luisada, 1978; Chen, 1959). Early investigators coined the term "dissociative anesthesia" to describe the PCP-induced state of altered consciousness in which higher brain functions seemed disconnected from awareness of the environment (Corssen, 1965). A significant number of patients suffered psychotic reactions during emergence from anesthesia. Oral PCP in subanesthetic doses proved able to control severe pain but also led to psychotic reactions (Griefenstein, 1958).

The psychotomimetic effects of PCP, noted in its earliest clinical trials, ranged from mild excitement to severe manic excitement and hallucinations (Vincent, 1979). Subanesthetic doses (0.1 mg/kg i.v.) induced body-image changes, feelings of estrangement, disorganization of thought, drowsiness and apathy in all subjects; feelings of inebriation, negativism, and hypnogogic states in a majority, and motor stereotypy in a large minority. The PCP-thought disorder included blocking echolalia, looseness of associations, neologisms and severe impairment of the capacity for abstraction; these are among the classical components of the schizophrenic syndrome. In this respect, PCP differs markedly from LSD and other hallucinogens which do not mimic the primary signs and symptoms of schizophrenia. The relationship between the analgesic, anesthetic, and psychotomimetic effects remains undetermined.

The question arises as to whether the diverse actions of PCP are mediated through interaction at specific receptor sites and whether these sites are related to the sites of action of other psychotomimetic drugs such as the opiate mixed agonist-antagonists. Preliminary studies by our laboratory (Zukin, 1979; 1981) and by others (Vincent, 1979) indicate that [^{3}H] PCP binds to specific sites in animal nervous tissue. Maayani and Weinstein (1980) had suggested that the filtration method might be unsuitable for detecting the pharmacologically relevant binding sites of [³H] PCP. More recently however, we (Zukin, 1981) and others (Vincent, 1980; Quirion, 1981; McQuinn, 1981) have shown this method applicable kinetically and in terms of specificity to the detection of PCP receptors. Moreover, Quirion et al (1981) have described essentially identical sites using both direct binding to slide-mounted brain sections and autoradiography.

Several pieces of evidence suggest that the sigma receptor and PCP binding site may be the same. Thus, of a large number of opiates tested, only cyclazocine-like opiates have been shown to displace [³H] PCP binding. Conversely, PCP and its derivatives can inhibit binding of [³H] cyclazocine to its lowest affinity (K_D = 70 nM) binding site. Behaviorally too the two classes of drugs can produce similar effects.

Recent animal-behavioral studies show that cyclazocine-like opiates display PCP-like properties. Teal and Holtzman (1980) proposed cyclazocine to possess both "opioid" and "nonopioid" properties based on their findings that the discriminative stimulus properties of the drug were only partially naloxone-reversible. In a subsequent discriminative stimulus study using rats trained to cyclazocine, Teal and Holtzman (1980) found that of twelve test compounds, ketocyclazocine, SKF-10,047, ethylketocyclazocine, PCP, ketamine, pentazocine, and levallorphan generalized to cyclazocine (the last two most weakly); morphine, nalorphine, amphetamine, mescaline, and LSD were inactive. Discriminative effects of cyclazocine were only partially reversible by naloxone. In a discriminative stimulus paradigm utilizing rats trained to PCP, Holtzman (1981) has found that animals trained to PCP generalized to cyclazocine, SKF-10,047 and cylorthan, whereas they do not generalize to nalorphine.

Thus, it would appear that opiates, much like adrenergic, cholinergic, and dopaminergic ligands, initiate their broad spectrum of diverse pharmacological actions by interaction with multiple receptor sites. It is interesting to note, on the one hand, the apparent complete cross-reactivity of μ and δ receptors. The finding that μ and δ sites exhibit differentiational sensitivity to GTP (Zukin, 1980; Pert, 1980) and the suggestion that they represent a single receptor in either a cyclase-coupled or uncoupled state (Gentleman et al, 1981) lend support to the concept that μ and δ receptors are functionally related in analogy to dopamine type 1 and type 2 receptors. In contrast, there is no such cross-reactivity between μ and either K or σ receptors. The failure of morphine and other "classical" opiates, including the narcotic antagonists naloxone and naltrexone, to bind substantially to K sites and at all to σ sites is of particular interest. Thus, it is intriguing to speculate that the σ receptors do not represent "opiate" receptors at all, but rather a unique class of sites at which a class of chemically diverse psychotomimetic drugs, including some of the opiates and PCP, produce their distinctive effects.

REFERENCES

Chang K-J, Cooper BR, Hazum E and Cuatrecasas P: Multiple opiate receptors: Different regional distribution in the brain and differential binding of opiates and opioid peptides. *Mol Pharmacol* 16:91–104, 1979

Chang K-J and Cuatrecasas P: Multiple opiate receptors; enkephalins and morphine bind to receptors of different specificity. *J Biol Chem* 254:2610–2618, 1979

Chang K-J, Hazum E and Cuatrecasas P: Possible role of distinct morphine and enkephaline receptors in mediating actions of benzomorphan drugs (putative K and σ receptors). *Proc Nat Acad Sci USA* 77:4469–4473, 1980

Chang K-J, Miller RJ and Cuatrecasus P: Interaction of enkephalin with opiate receptors in intact cultured cells. *Mol Pharmacol* 14:961–970, 1978

Chen G, Ensor CR, Russell D and Bohner B: The pharmacology of l-(l-phenylcyclohexyl) piperidine. HCl. *J Pharmacol Exp Ther* 127:241–250, 1959

Corssen G and Domino EF: Dissociative anesthesia: Further pharmacologic studies and first clinical experience with phencyclidine derivative Cl-581. *Anesth Analg* 45:29–40, 1965

Evans JM, Hogg MI, Lunn JN and Rosen M: Degree and duration by naloxone of effects of morphine in conscious subjects. *Br Med J* 2:589–591, 1974

Gilbert PE and Martin WR: The effects of morphine- and nalorphine-like drugs in the nondependent, morphine dependent and cyclazocine dependent chronic spinal dog. *J Pharmacol Exp Therap* 198:66–82, 1976

Goodman R, Snyder SH, Kuhar MJ and Young WS III: Differentiation of delta and mu opiate receptor localizations by light microscopic autoradiography. *Proc Nat Acad Sci USA* 77:6239–6243, 1980

Griefenstein FE, DeVault M, Yoshitake MD and Cajewski JE: A study of a l-arylcyclohexylamine for anesthesia. *Anesth Analg* 37:283–294, 1958

Haertzen CR: Subjective effects of narcotic antagonists cyclazocine and nalorphine on the addiction research center inventory (ARCI). *Psychopharmacologia* 18:366–377, 1970

Harris RA: Interactions between narcotic agonists, partial agonists and antagonists evaluated by schedule-controlled bheavior. *J Pharmacol Exp Ther* 213:497–503, 1980

Harris LS and Pierson AK: Some narcotic antagonists in the benzomorphan series. *J Pharmacol Exp Ther* 143:141–148, 1964

Hiller JM and Simon EJ: ³H-ethylketocyclazocine binding: Lack of evidence for a separate K receptor in rat CNS. *Eur J Pharmacol* 60:389–390, 1979

Holtzman SG: Narcotic antagonists as stimulants of behavior in the rat: Specific and nonspecific effects. In: MC Braude et al (eds.), *Narcotic Antagonists*. New York: Raven Press, pp 371–382, 1979

Holtzman SG: Phencyclidine-like discriminative effects of opioids in the rat. *J Pharmacol Exp Ther* 1981 (in press)

Holtzman SG and Jewett RE: Stimulation of behavior in the rat by cyclazocine: Effects of naloxone. *J Pharmacol Exp Ther* 187:380–390, 1973

Jasinski DR, Martin WR and Sapira JD: Antagonism of the subjective effects, behavioral, pupillary and respiratory depressant effects of cyclazocine by naloxone. *Clin Pharmacol Ther* 9:215–222, 1968

Keats AS and Telford J: RF Gould (ea.), *Narcotic Antagonists as Analgesics: Chemical Aspects in Molecular Modifications in Drug Design*. Washington, DC: American Chemical Society, 1964

Killam KF Jr, Brocco MJ and Robinson CA: Evaluation of narcotic and narcotic antagonist interactions in primates. *Ann NY Acad Sci* 281:331–335, 1976

Kosterlitz HW, Lord JAH, Paterson SJ and Waterfield AA: Effect of changes in the structure of enkephalins and of narcotic analgesic drugs on their interactions with μ- and δ-receptors. *Br J Pharmacol* 68:33–342, 1980

Kosterlitz HW and Paterson W: Characterization of opioid receptors in nervous tissue. *Proc R Soc Lond* 210:113–122, 1980

Kream RM and Zukin RS: Binding characteristics of a potent enkephalin analog. *Biochem Biophys Res Commun* 90:99–109, 1979

Lasagna L and Beecher HK: The analgesic effectiveness of nalorphine and nalorphine-morphine combinations in man. *J Pharmacol Exp Ther* 112:356–363, 1954

Leslie FM, Chavkin C and Cox BM: Ligand specificity of opioid binding sites in brain and peripheral tissues. In: EL Way (ed.), *Endogenous and Exogenous Opiate Agonists and Antagonists.* New York: Pergamon Press, pp 109–112, 1980

Lord JAH, Waterfield AA, Hughes J and Kosterlitz HW: Endogeneous opioid peptides: Multiple agonists and receptors. *Nature* 267:495–500, 1977

Lord JAH, Waterfield AA, Hughes J and Kosterlitz HW: HW Kosterlitz (ed.), *Multiple Opiate Receptors in Opiates and Endogenous Opioid Peptides.* Amsterdam: North-Holland Publishing, pp 275–280, 1976

Luisada PV: The phencyclidine psychosis: Phenomenology and treatment. In: RC Petersen and RC Stillman (eds.), *Phencylidine Abuse: An Appraisal.* NIDA Research Monograph 21, pp 241–253, 1978

Maayani S and Weinstein H: "Specific Binding" of ^{3}H-phencyclidine: Artifacts of the rapid filtration method. *Life Sci* 26:2011–2016, 1980

Martin WR: Opioid antagonists. *Pharmacol Review* 19:463–521, 1967

Martin WR, Eades CG, Thompson JA, Huppler RE and Gilbert PE: The effects of morphine and nalorphine-like drugs in the nondependent and morphine-dependent chronic spinal dog. *J Pharmacol Exp Therap* 197:517–532, 1976

Martin WR, Fraser HF, Gorodetzky CW and Rosenberg DE: Studies in the dependence producing potential of the narcotic antagonists 2-cyclopropylmethyl–2-dydroxy–5, 9 dimethyl–6,7 benzomorphan (cyclazocine, Win 20, 740, ARC II-C-3). *J Pharmacol Exp Therap* 150:426–436, 1965

Martin WR and Gorodetzky CW: Demonstration of tolerance to and physical dependence on N-allylnormorphine (nalorphine). *J Pharmacol Exp Therap* 150:437–442, 1965

McQuinn RL, Cone EJ, Shannon HE and Su T-P: Phencyclidine: I. Structure activity relationships of the cycloalkyl ring of phencyclidine. *J Med Chem* 1981 (in press)

Pasternak GW: Multiple opiate receptors: ^{3}H-ethylketocyclazocine receptor binding and ketocyclazocine analgesia. *Proc Nat Acad Sci USA* 77:3691–3694, 1980

Pert CB and Taylor D: EL Way (ed.), *Type 1 and Type 2 Opiate Receptors in Endogenous and Exogenous Opiate Agonists and Antagonists.* New York: Pergamon Press, pp 87–90, 1980

Quirion R, Hammer R. Herkenham M and Pert CB: A phencyclidine/sigma opiate receptor: Its visualization by tritium-sensitive film. *Proc Nat Acad Sci USA* 1981 (in press)

Robson LE and Kosterlitz HW: Specific protection of the binding sites of D-ala^2-D-leu^5-enkephalin (δ-receptors) and dihydromorphine (μ-receptors). *Proc R Soc Lond* 205:425–432, 1979

Roemer D, Buescher HH, Hill RC, Pless J, Bauer W, Cardinaux F, Closse A, Hauser D and Hyguenip R: A synthetic enzephalin analogue with prolonged parenteral and oral analgesic activity. *Nature* 268:547–549, 1977

Romer D, Buscher H, Hill RC, Maurer R, Petcher TJ, Welle HBA, Bakel HCCK and Akkerman AM: Bremazocine: A potent, long-acting opiate kappa agonist. *Life Sci* 27:971–978, 1980

Rosencrans JD, Chance WT and Spencer RM: The discriminative stimulus properties of cyclazocine: Generalization studies involving nalorphine, morphine and LSD. *Res Commun Chem Pathol Pharmacol* 20:221–237, 1978

Schaefer GJ and Holtzman SG: Discriminative effects of cyclazocine in the squirrel monkey. *J Pharmacol Exp Ther* 205:291–301, 1978

Simatov R, Childers SR and Snyder SH: The opiate receptor binding interaction of ^{3}H-methionine enkephalin: An opioid peptide. *Eur J Pharmacol* 47:319–331, 1978

Smith JR and Simon EJ: Selective protection of stereospecific enkephalin and opiate binding against inactivation by N-ethylmaleimide; evidence for two classes of opiate receptors. *Proc Nat Acad Sci USA* 77:281–284, 1980

Steinert HR, Holtzman SG and Jewett RE: Some agonistic actions of the morphine antagonist levallorphan on behavior and brain monoamines in the rat. *Psychopharmacologia* 31:35–46, 1973

Teal JJ and Holtzman SG: Discriminative stimulus effects of cyclazocine in the rat. *J Pharmacol Exp Ther* 212:368–376, 1980

Teal JJ and Holtzman SG: Discriminative stimulus effects of prototype opiate receptor agonists in monkeys. *Eur J Pharmacol* 68:1–10, 1980

Vincent JP, Kartalovski B, Geneste P, Kamenka JM and Lazdunski M: Interaction of phencyclidine ("angel dust") with a specific receptor in rat brain membranes. *Proc Nat Acad Sci USA* 76:4578–4682, 1979

Vincent J-P, Vignon J, Kartalovski B and Lazdunski M: Binding of phencyclidine to rat brain membranes: Technical aspects. *Eur J Pharmacol* 68:73–77, 1980

Vincent J-P, Vignon J, Kartalovski B and Lazdunski M: Compared properties of central and peripheral binding sites for phencyclidine. *Eur J Pharmacol* 68:79–82, 1980

Waterfield AA, Smokcum RWJ, Hughes J, Kosterlitz HW and Henderson G: In vitro pharmacology of the opioid peptides, enkephalins and endorphins. *Eur J Pharmacol* 43:107–116, 1977

Wray SR: A correlative evaluation of cyclazocine, LSD and naloxone on continuous discriminated avoidance in rats. *Psychopharmacologia* 26:29–43, 1972

Zukin RS and Gintzler AR: Guanyl nucleotide interactions with opiate receptors in guinea pig brain and ileum. *Brain Res* 186:486–491, 1980

Zukin SR, Margolis A and Zukin RS: Biochemical Evidence for Kappa and Sigma Receptors. 1981 (in preparation)

Zukin RS and Zukin SR: Demonstration of ^{3}H-cyclazocine binding to multiple opiate receptor sites. *Mol Pharm* 1981 (in press)

Zukin SR and Zukin RS: Identification and characterization of ^{3}H-phencyclidine binding to specific brain receptor sites in PCP. In: E Domino (ed.), *Historical and Current Perspectives.* Ann Arbor: NPP Books, 1981

Zukin SR and Zukin RS: Specific [^{3}H] pencyclidine binding in rat central nervous system. *Proc Nat Acad Sci USA* 76:5372–5376, 1979

9

Behavioral Factors in Drug Dependence and Withdrawal: A Discussion

STEVEN M. MIRIN

A considerable body of clinical and laboratory data suggest that behavioral factors, including both classical and operant conditioning, play an important role in the development and maintenance of drug dependence. This discussion will focus on some of the major contributions of behavioral research in this area as illustrated by the papers we have just heard. Since much of this work has been carried out in opiate users, I will, for the sake of clarity and consistency, focus on this particular area, bearing in mind the potential application of these findings to other forms of substance abuse.

CONDITIONED RESPONDING IN OPIATE USERS

The role of conditioning factors in opiate dependence and withdrawal has been explored by a number of research groups (Wikler, 1968; O'Brien, 1981) including our own (Meyer, 1979). In the course of such studies it has been noted that under certain circumstances, addicts will respond to the mere anticipation of drug effects or to an injection of saline as if they had actually received an opiate drug. In our own studies (Meyer, 1979) addicts pretreated with a narcotic antagonist like naltrexone will exhibit such responses (ie, constricted pupils, diminished respirations, feelings of euphoria) when exposed to subsequent injections of "blocked" heroin. O'Brien's group has made similar observations, as illustrated by the data presented here today (O'Brien, 1981).

The role of such conditioned responses in the perpetuation of drug dependence has been the subject of considerable speculation. Our own observation has been that individuals who manifest conditioned opioid-like responses to injections of "blocked" heroin also report relatively high levels of drug craving, even after conditioned responding to blocked heroin is no longer evident. Consistent with this observation they also tend to relapse more readily when discharged into the community, suggesting that conditioned responding to drug-related stimuli may be a poor prognostic sign in this population.

Another important finding of behavioral research in the addictions is the observation by Wikler (1968) that rats previously addicted to morphine will exhibit "wet dog shakes", a sign of morphine abstinence, when placed in an environment in which they had previously experienced morphine addiction and withdrawal. Similarly, in individuals with a history of opiate dependence such conditioned abstinence responses may be elicited by stimuli previously associated with opiate intoxication or withdrawal. For example, ex-addicts and patients on methadone will exhibit conditioned abstinence symptoms when shown pictures of other addicts "shooting up", drug paraphrenalia, etc. These symptoms are indistinguishable from those produced by narcotic withdrawal (O'Brien, 1974).

The observation of conditioned abstinence phenomena in both animals and man has led to speculation about the role of such responses in the genesis of relapse. In our own experience (Mirin, 1974) conditioned abstinence phenomena are characteristically accompanied by increased drug craving and drug seeking behavior. Where such behavior culminates in the experience of drug related (ie, pharmacologic) reinforcement a powerful link has been forged in the behavioral chain leading to relapse. In this context Wikler (1973) has postulated that effective blockade of opiate reinforcement should result in the eventual extinction of opiate using behavior. Though clearly applicable to animal models of addiction (Carnathan, 1977) this process has yet to be demonstrated in man.

A number of laboratories have attempted to test the extinction hypothesis under controlled conditions. In an earlier study by O'Brien and associates (1974), addicts pre-treated with the narcotic antagonist cyclazocine were allowed to self-administer hydromorphone (Dilaudid) or saline under double-blind conditions. Initially, injection of either substance was followed by subjective reports of euphoria. In most subjects, this conditioned response quickly extinguished; in a few, however, conditioned responding to "blocked" injections of hydromorphone was maintained. In our own studies (Meyer, 1979), ex-addicts pretreated with naltrexone were allowed to self-administer increasing doses of intravenous heroin. About half discontinued opiate use after three or four unsuccessful attempts at "getting high." In these subjects the decision to discontinue heroin challenges of antagonist blockade seemed more consistent with a process of cognitive labeling (ie, that heroin was really "unavailable") than extinction in the classical sense.

A second group of naltrexone-treated individuals persisted in self-administering heroin ($\bar{x}$ = 15 trials) despite antagonist blockade of opiate effects. Interestingly, it was this group that manifested conditioned autonomic responses (ie, pupillary constriction, diminished respiratory rate) and euphoria after injecting "blocked" heroin. Compared to those subjects who stopped challenging antagonist blockade after only a few trials, they also reported relatively high levels of drug craving, even after heroin was no longer available to them.

The practical implication of those findings were subsequently explored in our follow up studies (Meyer, 1979) where we found that in the month after discharge the rate of relapse to heroin use was much higher among those who manifested conditioned autonomic responses to blocked heroin. Thus, one might reasonably speculate that in the course of maintaining an addiction some addicts develop a particular responsiveness to conditioned stimuli which signal increased drug availability. These stimuli, in turn, trigger a rise in drug craving and drug seeking behavior. On the research ward this propensity is manifested by prolonged challenging of antagonist blockade. In the community it is expressed by a high rate of drop out from antagonist treatment and subsequent relapse to heroin use.

SCHEDULE EFFECTS ON DRUG USING BEHAVIOR

A relatively neglected area of behavioral research involves the role of schedule effects in the development and maintenance of drug taking behavior. The work of both Dews (1981) and Stollerman (1981) suggests that, at least in animals, drug seeking behavior may be profoundly influenced by factors specific to the relationship between the behavior itself and the delivery (ie, schedule) of reinforcement. Our own, albeit less rigorous, observations (Meyer, 1979) suggest that scheduling may also effect drug seeking behavior in man. For example, addicts working for heroin made available on a fixed interval (FI) schedule will perform such work in a pattern reminiscent of FI responding in animal studies. Work output (in this case, lever pulling) characteristically increased just prior to the "purchase" of each heroin dose. Moreover, this pattern of responding was maintained whether subjects waited two, four, or six hours between each injection (Meyer, 1979).

In contrast, addicts "on the street" usually experience opiate reinforcement on an uncertain (ie, variable interval) schedule. The effect of this schedule on operant responding (ie, hustling behavior) is to assure that such behavior is more or less continuous, declining only in the immediate post injection period.

Finally, lest we adhere too closely to a behavioral focus, Dr. Mulé's (1981) paper reminds us that, in man, drug seeking behavior is also shaped by the psychosocial and biological context in which it occurs. Indeed, even the consumption of a powerful reinforcer like heroin is influenced by the drug-using behavior of one's peers. Thus, in our subjects who were allowed to get high on heroin, the frequency of drug self-administration (ie, q2h, q4h or q6h) for each individual was clearly influenced by the drug using behavior of their intoxicated peers.

To summarize, behavioral studies of the type presented here today have shed considerable light on a very complex area. Though at first glance drug-using behavior appears to be under conscious control, it is subtly, but clearly, shaped by behavioral contingencies. Opiate addiction, like the other so-called "volitional" disorders, develops in the context of a series of voluntary choices. Once a repetitive pattern of drug use is established, however, this behavior is clearly shaped by a host of other factors, including conditioned responding, schedule effects, and factors particular to the psychosocial milieu in which drug consumption and reinforcement takes place. It is these commonalities which link the various addictive disorders and make them so difficult to treat. Hopefully, the insights provided by behavioral research will provide a foundation upon which effective treatment strategies may be based.

REFERENCES

Carnathan G, Meyer RE and Cochin J: Narcotic blockade, length of addiction and persistence of intravenous morphine self-administration in rats. *Psychopharmacology* 54:67-71, 1977

Dews PB: Maintenance of behavior by "schedules": An unfamiliar contributor to the maintenance of the abuse. Presented at a Symposium of the International Anti-Drug Abuse Foundation, April 1981

Meyer RE and Mirin SM: Operant analysis. In: RE Meyer and SM Mirin (eds.), *The Heroin Stimulus*. New York: Plenum Press, pp 61-91, 1979

Meyer RE, Mirin SM and Zackon F: Community outcome on narcotic antagonists. In: RE Meyer and SM Mirin (eds.), *The Heroin Stimulus*. New York: Plenum Press, pp 215-230, 1979

Mirin, SM: A multimodality approach to opiate addiction. *Psych Opin* 11:35-42, 1974

Mule SJ: Behavior in excess: An examination of the volitional disorders. Presented at a Symposium of the International Anti-Drug Abuse Foundation, April 1981

O'Brien CP: The effects of conditioning on human opiate addicts. Presented at a Symposium of the International Anti-Drug Abuse Foundation, April 1981

O'Brien CP, Chaddock B, Woody G and Greenstein R: Systematic extinction of addiction associated rituals using narcotic antagonists. Presented in part at the American Psychosomatic Society Annual Meeting, March 1974

Stolerman IP: Behavioral analysis of drug taking and drug dependence. Presented at a Symposium of the International Anti-Drug Abuse Foundation, April 1981

Wikler A: Dynamics of drug dependence: Implications of a conditioning theory for research and treatment. *Arch Gen Psychiatry* 28:611-616, 1973

Wikler A: Interaction of physical dependence and conditioning. *A Res Nerv and Mental Disorders Proc* 46:280-287, 1968

10

Epidemiology of the Current Heroin Crisis

BLANCHE FRANK
DOUGLAS S. LIPTON

The New York State Division of Substance Abuse Services is mandated to assess the problem of drug abuse in the state—to determine its magnitude, its trends, the drugs of choice, the populations-at-risk, and the development of incipient epidemics. Consequently, the agency has a strong commitment to an epidemiologic study of the drug abuse problem.

I want to describe for you the everyday work of the epidemiology section of the agency, and then to describe the way in which we tracked the current heroin crisis in the state.

Our epidemiology section is divided into three units which reflect the three research strategies we use—the indirect indicator unit, the direct survey unit, and the ethnography or street studies unit.

The indirect indicator unit gathers data from a variety of official sources Included among these data are drug-related arrests, drug-related emergency room episodes, cases of serum hepatitis, drug-related deaths, and admissions to drug treatment programs. Although the exact nature of the association between drug abuse and these indicators is not known, they are thought to reflect changes in drug use trends.

Each of the indicators is confounded by many problems: problems associated with the policies of the agencies that do the data collecting; problems associated with the vagaries and vicissitudes of data collection; and problems intrinsic to the indicators, irrespective of policy decisions and data collection. Epidemiologically, each indicator is only an imperfect reflection of the drug problem. If, however, most of the indicators point in the same direction and follow a similar trend over time, there is strong evidence that the problem is increasing or decreasing.

The direct survey unit, unlike the indirect indicator unit, generates its own data through the conduct of population surveys and does not rely on data generated by other agencies. Also, unlike the indicator unit that primarily analyzes trends, the survey unit can estimate incidence and prevalence of drug abuse. For instance, school children (in the 7th through 12th grades) a population particularly at risk of drug abuse, were randomly sampled and surveyed using a questionnaire that was self-administered. The results were statistically weighted and projected to the total population of school children in the 7th through the 12th grades in New York State to give an estimate of drug abusers in that population. Currently, the unit is supervising a computer-directed telephone survey of household residents in the state. The survey inquires into the use of a variety of drugs; the frequency, recency, and intensity of use; age at first use; and dysfunctionalities associated with use. The findings from the carefully selected sample will be weighted and projected to the total household population. Thus, estimates of drug abusers among the household population will be calculated.

Direct population surveys, however, like indirect indicators, have their shortcomings. First, surveys are useful in describing the characteristics of a large population. When, however, a rare behavior is studied, such as drug abuse, it is necessary to sample a very large population, and perhaps over-sample segments of the population having the highest use rates in order to achieve statistical reliability. This, in turn, increases the cost, making this research strategy considerably more expensive than the others. Furthermore, surveys cannot measure actual drug activity; they can only collect self-reports of recalled past action or of prospective action. Many respondents hesitate to give completely candid information about behavior that is so stigmatized. Finally, we know that direct surveys are not helpful in determining the prevalence of heroin abuse. The heroin-abusing segments of the population usually do not surface in school surveys and traditional household surveys, and if they do, they are probably unlikely to report their heroin use.

Finally, there is the street studies unit. In order to get timely data and knowledge of current drug use and availability, it is often necessary to study drug activity in the field and in its natural habitat. Consequently, the members of the street studies unit regularly observe the availability and prices of drugs sold in the "street"—on the illicit market. These workers are themselves former drug users who are knowledgeable about the behavior they observe and who physically resemble the population engaged in drug activity. Occasionally, the field workers try to engage in conversation with dealers, buyers, and onlookers to gather more information about use patterns and shifts in use.

In addition, the field unit has selected a sample of secondary schools that its members observe and monitor twice a year so that changes may be determined in any drug activity that may exist outside the school among the school-aged children. When special situations develop, the field unit is often asked to explore the situation by observing the scene. For instance, a newspaper article carried a story about teenage drug dealing in Manhattan. The field unit was asked to study several areas in the city to determine the extent of teenage drug dealing.

Street studies, like indirect indicators and direct surveys, have their weaknesses. The informal sampling and uncertain representativeness of the observations are shortcomings in themselves. It is not clear how far-reaching and how generalizable the findings are. An additional weakness is the danger involved in being a mere observer: since the field workers do not engage in drug using or dealings, and their identities as researchers are not revealed, their presence in these areas is often difficult to justify to those participating in the drug subculture.

Thus, given our three units and the research strategies they use and the limitations in each, we proceed very cautiously by using at least two of the strategies in assessing particular drug activity. In the literature of social research, the use of several research strategies in the study of a problem is called "triangulation." One sees our attempt at this approach when the heroin problem began to escalate in New York City in 1979.

For several years during the middle of the 1970s, heroin activity seemed to be declining. Trends in indirect indicators of heroin use were going down, the street studies unit found diminished availability, and the direct surveys were certainly not finding heroin use among respondents. In fact, the state agency was devoting more and more of its energy to combating illicit non-narcotic drug abuse and prescription drug misuse.

In the middle of 1979, the street studies unit was bringing back the word that more white heroin than the Mexican brown heroin was appearing on the streets, and that dealers in Harlem were talking glowingly of the purity of newly available heroin.

In 1979 we carefully watched the indicators. By the third quarter of 1979, some interesting trends started to develop. Readmissions to methadone programs in New York City had been declining steadily since 1975 to a low point in 1978. In the first three quarters of 1979, however, readmissions to New York's methadone programs started to increase. In fact they increased 22 percent over the comparable period in 1978. Similarly, the percentage of morphine positive urine samples among methadone clients doubled from early 1979 to the middle of 1979—from two percent to four percent of the samples. Thus, the indicators gave us some interesting clues, that addicts were returning to treatment, that heroin was probably the drug of abuse, and that those in methadone treatment were also abusing heroin.

By the end of 1979, when other indirect indicator data were available, the trend was unmistakable in New York City. Between 1978 and 1979:

- opiate-involved felony arrests in New York City showed an increase of nine percent (from 4,123 to 4,503);
- heroin emergency room episodes reported for a sample of New York SMSA hospitals increased 49 percent (from 480 to 713);
- deaths due to intravenous narcotism increased 92 percent (from 246 to 472); and
- treatment admissions with heroin as the primary drug of abuse increased 26 percent (from 18,644 to 23,464).

At the beginning of 1980, the street studies unit conducted interviews with 150 heroin users and/or dealers in 30 locations in New York City. The responses indicated that the quality of the heroin was excellent. Many informants compared it to the heroin of the past: "The stuff out there is like the O.D. bags of the sixties." "The shit is so good it makes you think you are back in the days." Furthermore the purity was so high that a series of dealers were able to dilute the heroin many times and still preserve the "kick." Some dealers said:

"I got it man, I got the real deal. I can give you a good play on some pure (ie, unadulterated heroin). This is on a fifteen (ie, can be diluted 15 to one and still have strength)". "So now I give it a 20 or a 22 and sell it for pure; they can put a five or a three on it and still get over."

The dealers and users recognized the fact that it was heroin coming from a new source—Southwest Asia. For instance, this dialogue was reported:

"Wow I haven't seen or heard of that kind of shit in years."
"Well my people got it man. Straight off the boat."
"I wonder where it comes from?"
"Man I think its from Iran! Yep Iran man!"

During 1980 we continued to track the indicators, our field unit continued to observe the street, and we kept alerting the executive managers of our agency to the findings. But, given the vagaries and vicissitudes of data collection, there were some changes in indicators. For instance, readmissions to methadone treatment programs were no longer available since that methadone registry ceased to exist and another registry started up, which lost the distinction between new admissions and readmissions. The sample of consistently reporting hospital emergency rooms changed somewhat, and a new trend was established. Nevertheless, the increasing trend in heroin activity in New York City was generally more pronounced in 1980 than it was in 1979. Between 1979 and 1980:

- heroin admissions to emergency rooms increased 82 percent (from 1,924 to 3,494);

- preliminary numbers of deaths due to intravenous narcotism showed a 33 percent increase (472 to 630);
- cases of serum hepatitis B+, which is considered an indicator of incidence or new use of intravenous drug use and which had remained stable between 1978 and 1979, increased 18 percent from 1979 to 1980 (487 to 577);
- admissions of inmates to the detoxification program on Riker's Island also had remained relatively stable between 1978 and 1979, but rose 34 percent between 1979 and 1980 (from 7,239 to 9,704);
- the Drug Enforcement Administration in its studies of purity of street samples found relative consistency of three percent in Harlem, but an increase from 8.5 percent to 12.6 percent for street bags on the Lower East Side;
- finally, heroin treatment admissions, rather than increase, declined 10 percent (from 23,464 to 21,107), simply because treatment programs could not accommodate additional clients. By the end of 1980, waiting lists existed in methadone maintenance programs, residential drug-free and ambulatory detoxification programs. Currently, the waiting lists number more than 1,000 names.

Again, the street studies unit brought back its reports. Heroin dealing was taking place throughout the city and street bags were averaging about $10 per bag. What was most disconcerting was their finding that six or seven dealers were selling heroin for $4 per bag, a price that was unheard of since the 1960s. Coupled with the high purity found on the Lower East Side, there findings signaled a very serious problem.

Thus, from indirect indicators and street observation, we have had a close watch on the current heroin situation. Perhaps a look at the epidemiologic triad of agent, environment and host can shed some additional light.

First, the "agent." What has exacerbated the current heroin problem is the increased availability of heroin in the last few years, chiefly from Southwest Asia. In 1979, the US Drug Enforcement Administration estimated that the opium cultivation in the world was almost 1,800 metric tons. This volume can be best appreciated when it is compared to the volume produced during the heroin epidemic years of the 1960s and early 1970s. At that time an annual production of only about 80 metric tons of opium from Turkey was responsible for the heroin traffic to the United States. Although not all the current opium produced in the world will find its way to the United States, opium cultivation is considerable, it will find its way to where the profits are the greatest, and it is produced in countries with which diplomatic relations are extremely strained (Iran and Afghanistan). Furthermore, the DEA expects production levels to remain high through 1981, somewhat diminished in Southwest Asia but increased in Southeast Asia or the Golden Triangle countries of Thailand, Burma, and Laos.

Another important consideration is the fact that opium cultivation is only the first step in an already well-developed operation. Raw opium is converted to morphine base in clandestine laboratories in Middle Eastern countries and converted to heroin principally in French and Italian laboratories. The laboratories of the "French Connection" days are back in business once again, in the hands of very experienced entrepreneurs who have renewed old Mafia connections in the United States. Thus, the experience of the past has quickly made this a well-coordinated operation put in place fairly easily and very effectively.

A final comment about the "agent" concerns the way heroin is currently used. Although heroin is usually injected, the media carries news of how heroin is now being snorted and smoked. Little is known about the consequences of this form of use, although we know that the major problem of addiction in Asia was opium smoking. Nevertheless, the smoking of marijuana and the snorting of cocaine have become socially more acceptable and less stigmatized in this country. It is conceivable that the smoking and snorting of heroin may also gain wider acceptance among the vastly larger number of marijuana and cocaine users.

As for the "environment," this country's heroin problem tends to concentrate in northeastern cities, such as New York, Newark, Philadelphia, and Washington, although it is reported in Detroit and Phoenix as well. Unlike the late 1960s and early 1970s when large metropolitan areas throughout the United States had to deal with increased heroin activity, the current problem seems to be contained in several cities. A few reasons are offered for the very different pattern of distribution. The Drug Enforcement Administration believes that Mafia connections and the networks of independent entrepreneurs are so well-established in the New York-Washington region that there is no need to go elsewhere. Furthermore, the demand is greatest in New York City. In fact, it is still believed that half the addicts in the United States reside in New York City. Second, other regions have their special drug interests. For instance, Miami is dominated by cocaine traffic. Heroin traffickers may not even want to challenge the cocaine interests. In Chicago and the midwest, the Mexican heroin interests tend to dominate. Although Mexican heroin has diminished in availability, that criminal network may exert enough influence to prevent other heroin from entering. These well established dealing and criminal networks can distribute heroin if and when supplies are obtained.

Although these conjectures cannot be verified, the fact remains that during the two years that the heroin problem has increased, heroin availability seems to be confined to the northeastern corridor. The implications of the current situation—unlike the situation several years ago—are that those who are interested in heroin would have to migrate to the places where heroin is available and would therefore be attracted to the northeastern region of the country. In past years, the supply would follow the demand, today the situation might be quire different. Again this is in the realm of conjecture.

As for the "host," the distinguishing characteristic of current heroin abusers is their age. From emergency room data, treatment admissions, death data, it appears that the addicts currently most visible are those over the age of 30. Many of these are probably former addicts who have been lured back by the white heroin; some probably had been using all along but the heroin now available may have brought their use to dysfunctional levels. Whatever the pattern, many of these users have already had an immediate and overwhelming impact on the treatment system.

We expect, however, a second wave of users to impact the treatment system. These are the new abusers. The usual history of heroin addiction shows that it takes a year to two years (what is euphemistically called the "honeymoon" period) before the addict surfaces in treatment. We may have begun to see these users surfacing in the criminal justice system among adolescent inmates in New York City admitted to the detoxification program on Riker's Island and in the health system in the recent increase in cases of serum hepatitis B+.

There may even be a third wave of abusers who will be seeking treatment, those who start by snorting and smoking heroin and whose addiction histories may take a longer time to develop.

In any case the overall epidemiologic implications of the current heroin crisis are grave and the solutions require considerable resources on the local, state, federal and international levels in terms of increased treatment capability, more effective law enforcement, more effective programs in prevention, and, *surely,* strategic diplomacy at the international level.

We in the epidemiology section will continue to do our monitoring. We look forward to the time when we may report to you that the trends are declining and the crisis has passed.

11

Empirical Patterns of Heroin Consumption Among Selected Street Heroin Users

BRUCE D. JOHNSON

What are street heroin users really like? This question has perplexed policy makers for several years and is likely to do so in the near future as well. The public image holds that the addict is so physically dependent upon heroin that this drug must be injected several times per day and in large quantities or else the person will become severely sick. In order to obtain the heroin, the user must generally resort to crime to finance this habit; habit sizes of $100 per day or more are claimed by many heroin users and believed to be typical by the public.

This widely believed public image of the heroin addict has been hard to locate, however. National surveys of the adult and youth population show that low proportions have ever used heroin, and generally under half a percentage point have used it on a weekly or more regular basis (Miller and Cisin, 1980; Johnston et al, 1979; O'Donnell et al, 1976). Robins' (1973, 1974) study of Vietnam veterans showed that the vast majority of soldiers who reported physical dependence in Vietnam did not return to heroin use upon return to the U.S. The research of Zinberg and Harding (1979; Zinberg, 1979) demonstrate patterns of what they call "controlled heroin use" among subjects who report previous physical dependence.

McAuliffe and Gordon (1974, 1975, 1979, 1980) also raise questions about the importance of physical dependence as a necessary condition for 'addiction.' According to McAuliffe and Gordon's (1980) theory of reinforcement and combination of effects:

> there are important disadvantages associated with equating addiction with physical dependence as laymen do . . . (since this idea) encourages the seriously misleading impression . . . that a user is

relatively safe as long as physical dependence is avoided (p 139). In the long term addict, euphoria, withdrawal symptoms, and other miscellaneous reinforcing effects combine in various proportions to yield a complex schedule of reinforcement that sustains continued use. The exact weighting of each effect . . . may vary from time to time within a given individual and from addict to addict. . . . Street addicts who are sick from withdrawal and have only maintenance doses on hand are obviously satisfied to respond to just one component. . . . With a larger supply, they typically respond . . . by reducing sickness and enjoying euphoric effects, too. . . . At any given time, most street addicts are distributed in intermediate positions, where they avoid withdrawal and receive intermittent positive rewards. *It is the history of reinforcement gained from using drugs in all these ways that accounts for an individual's drug derived motivation for opiate use.* (p 349).

This paper is narrowly focused upon describing the heroin consuming behavior of a few selected heroin users. No particular theoretical position is advanced or "tested," since the data were not originally collected to test theories of physical dependence and addiction, nor were subjects selected as representative of any population. Rather, the following brief portraits of loves of several subjects provides new insights about the stability (or lack thereof) in patterns of heroin consumption. These patterns, however, raise questions relevant to theories of addiction which will be alluded to, but not resolved in this paper. Through careful description and analysis of behavior patterns, day-by-day, of several persons who exhibit continuing patterns of heroin consumption, a better understanding of how heroin is used, sought, purchased, and distributed will emerge. This will contribute to an improved model of the addiction process which must be developed in the future.

METHODOLOGY

The data come from two pilot-study years (1978–79) of a long-term effort to study the economic behavior of opiate users and street hustlers. The original design was to locate research subjects who exhibited differing criminal and drug use patterns; only those subjects who used heroin during a 30 day period are considered in this paper. Nonheroin users (all injected cocaine) and subjects enrolled in methadone treatment are not discussed in this paper. The intent was to maximize intersubject variation rather than select a representative sample. This means that the subjects should not be considered as a "sample" as that term is ordinarily used in statistics, nor representative of any larger population. The term "study group" will be applied to the subjects whose crime and heroin/drug use is analyzed here.

The research team established a field station in a well-known ghetto neighborhood in New York City. Subjects were recruited by professional ethnographic staff and trained ex-addict fieldworkers. They reported to the storefront field office where they were interviewed for 30 or more consecutive days. A daily interview instrument was administered and data was collected on the respondent's involvement and cash returns from several crimes, the type and dollar amount of drugs used, their income from all sources, and their expenditures for all purposes during the preceding day. Respondents were paid a modest sum for their time and information.

The characteristics of the 31 respondents were compared with clients attending public methadone clinics in East Harlem. A majority of both the study group and MMTP clients were over age 30, but the study group had a substantially lower proportion of females than the clinics. The ethnic distributions are relatively similar except that blacks are proportionately larger in the study group. The group exhibited extensive patterns of drug use and crime. Over 90 percent had been arrested, and 80 percent had been incarcarated. Their educational level was low, only a third had graduated from high school and only 6 percent were employed at the point of the daily interviews. The subjects exhibited long term patterns of heroin use, routine cocaine consumption, and extensive criminal careers as measured by arrests and incarcerations. All were chronic users of heroin or cocaine, which they generally consumed by injection.

Before presenting the data from the heroin-using subjects, several caveats may be noted. These data were obtained in 1978 and 1979 in a small neighborhood in one of the New York City's highest addiction communities. Existing evidence (Frank, 1979, 1980) suggests that the quality of street heroin and the severity of the heroin problem was at about its lowest point in the 1970 decade during these two years. Thus, even persons who used heroin several times daily may have been consuming so little heroin or opiate equivalent that they were not physically dependent in the classical definition of this phenomena. This research effort was never intented, nor is it currently attempting, to measure directly various socio-psycho-physiological states of these respondents such as degree of withdrawal sickness, desire for euphoria, perceptions of tolerance or craving, etc; so the number of days of nonheroin/nonopiate use and dollar amounts used below provides imprecise and faulty indicators of such concepts. The portraits of several types of heroin users will give a better "feel" about the diversity in heroin consumption patterns and raise important questions without proving or disproving particular hypotheses about addiction.

EMPIRICAL PATTERNS OF HEROIN CONSUMPTION

The data show considerable variation in heroin use patterns. One of the striking findings is that many chronic heroin users exhibit several days of nonheroin use during the 30 day period. Even among the subjects who used heroin most regularly (see next paragraph), all except one respondent exhibited days of nonheroin use.

In an attempt to develop a simple distinction between "addicts" and "nonaddicts," several typologies of respondents were studied. The most empirically useful classification was the proportion of 30 consecutive days that the subject used heroin. Thus, respondents were classified according to a *Regularity of Heroin Use Typology:* (1) "Near daily" users (n=9) consumed heroin 75 percent or more of the days; these subjects used heroin on an average of 27 (90 percent of 30) days. (2) "Regular" users (n=16) consumed heroin on 40–74 percent of their 30 days; they used heroin on an average of 18 (60 percent of 30) days. (3) "Irregular" heroin users (n=6) had up to 40 percent of days with use; but actually used it on only about two (7 percent of 30) days. Thus, the image of the daily heroin user, which is widely accepted in the professional literature and assumed by the press and lay public, was not evidenced by most of the study's subjects.

Moreover, among all heroin users, extensive variation in heroin consumption occurs. Important differences in heroin consumption occurs as the regularity of heroin use increases. The irregular heroin users use heroin on less than 10 percent of all days. Even on days of heroin use, they consume more than $20 on less than a quarter of these days. In short, they seldom use heroin, and in small amounts if they do. The regular heroin users consume over $20 on about two fifths of the days with a mean* consumption of $23. The near daily heroin users, however, consume heroin on an average of 90 percent of the days; they use over $20 on almost three quarters of their use days. Their mean consumption on days of heroin use in $43. In short, the near daily heroin users appear to have characteristics (many days of use, with large amounts consumed per day of use) associated with physical dependence.

Thus, to the extent that the regularity and amount of heroin consumed is indicative of physical dependence, the near daily heroin users most closely approximate this condition. The regular heroin users provide much less compelling evidence of possible physical dependence to heroin while the irregular heroin users appear not to be dependent regardless of how far this

---

*The arithmetic mean on days of use is used here. The median is somewhat less. Standards deviations are large relative to the mean—as expected given the selection process.

concept is stretched. Several days of nonheroin consumption are partially accounted for by consumption of methadone, both licit and illicit; but many subjects still exhibit several days without any opiate use as the following case histories show.

CASE HISTORIES OF HEROIN CONSUMPTION FOR SELECTED RESPONDENTS: HOW STABLE ARE PATTERNS OF HEROIN USE DAY-BY-DAY?

The following case history material offer additional insight about respondents exhibiting different patterns of heroin consumption during the study period. The emergent finding is that each respondent consumes relatively differing amounts of heroin on consecutive days. The cases represent different patterns of heroin use.

Theo W, Sonny C, and Stephen H were three of the nine near-daily heroin users. Theo W was a very successful burglar who used large amounts of heroin. Sonny C was a street drug dealer, specializing in heroin sales. Stephen H was the one subject who used (and continues) to use heroin every single day; he also happens to be a versatile and successful criminal. Frenchy S was one of the most frequent heroin users among respondents classified as "regular" users; his heroin consumption on days of use is somewhat higher than the mean among those in the regular heroin use category. He also used illicit methadone several times during the daily interviews and joined a MMTP program during later interviews. Bobby H used heroin on as many days as Frenchy S but has an average consumption that was very low. Vance D was among the least frequent "regular" heroin users; he seldom exhibits successive days of use. Ulric Q is a former methadone patient who is an "irregular" heroin user, more regular cocaine user, and a severe alcoholic.

A brief biographical portrait of each is provided. Information about each subject's pattern of economic support as well as his day-by-day heroin consumption and methadone use is provided from life history interviews and the daily interview forms.

In the graphs presented for each subject, the vertical axis contains the dollar amount of heroin used on a given day. The horizontal axis is the number of the day after the first interview; no specific calendar days are given to protect the respondent's anonymity. The "X" on some charts indicates use of illicit methadone, the height of the X indicates the dollar amount paid for such illicit methadone (the amount in mgs could not be obtained). On Sonny C's graph (2), the small circles "o" indicate that he consumed methadone given at a detoxification program; the height of the circle indicates the amount of heroin he also consumed on that same day.

Theo W

Theo W is a black male about 50 years old. He is one of two professional burglars in the study group who uses a large amount of heroin and
cocaine when he has a high income. Although he has worked at odd jobs in
the recent past, he has been a lifelong criminal.

He has spent almost half his life in prison. He was first arrested for
robbery at age 14 and sent to the State Training School on two different
occasions. On an adult robbery charge, he was sentenced to 25–30 years,
but served eleven in state prison, mainly in the 1960s. Although arrested
subsequently, he has managed to avoid long prison sentences.

He first started using heroin in 1948–49, and has been mainlining heroin
most of the time he was not in prison. He was asked: "How much are you
spending now?"

"It's difficult to put a value on it now. Because you can get like a ten
dollar bag, or a half of a quarter or a $50 quarter." When asked whether
addicted or not: "I'd say I've got a chippy, but the way narcotics are today,
it's nothing worse than the flu really" (but admitted to being addicted now
when asked directly).

He was one of the few subjects with several days where he used $100
of heroin (but never more) even though he had more cash from successful
burglaries on several of those days. His heroin use profile (Fig. 1) is very
ragged, indicating many days of nonheroin use preceded and followed by
days of use up to $100. On six of these nonuse days, however, he purchased
street methadone which he felt held him over to the next day. On two days
(26 and 34), he used no opiate; on both of the previous days, he had either
used methadone or a low amount ($20) of heroin.

Although not shown on the graph, Theo W used an sizable amount of
cocaine on days when he also used heroin, generally when he had a large
income from a successful burglary. He also drinks heavily. "I was in the
hospital about three times for drinking. . . . Twice it was for what they called
acute pancreatitis, and then one time I went for detox. . . . I used to run up
a bill at the liquor store of over $100 in a two week period." Despite his
irregular use of street methadone, he has never been on a methadone program
although he was once in a detoxification program.

Sonny C

Sonny C is a black male who basically supports himself by being a street
heroin dealer. He began using heroin in the late 1950s and was quite active
in the following years, although there were some years with irregular use.

He has not escaped the arms of the law. He recalls about 14 arrests,
mainly for possession of heroin or sale of methadone. He has served about 5
years in prison, the longest was a three year stint for a robbery.

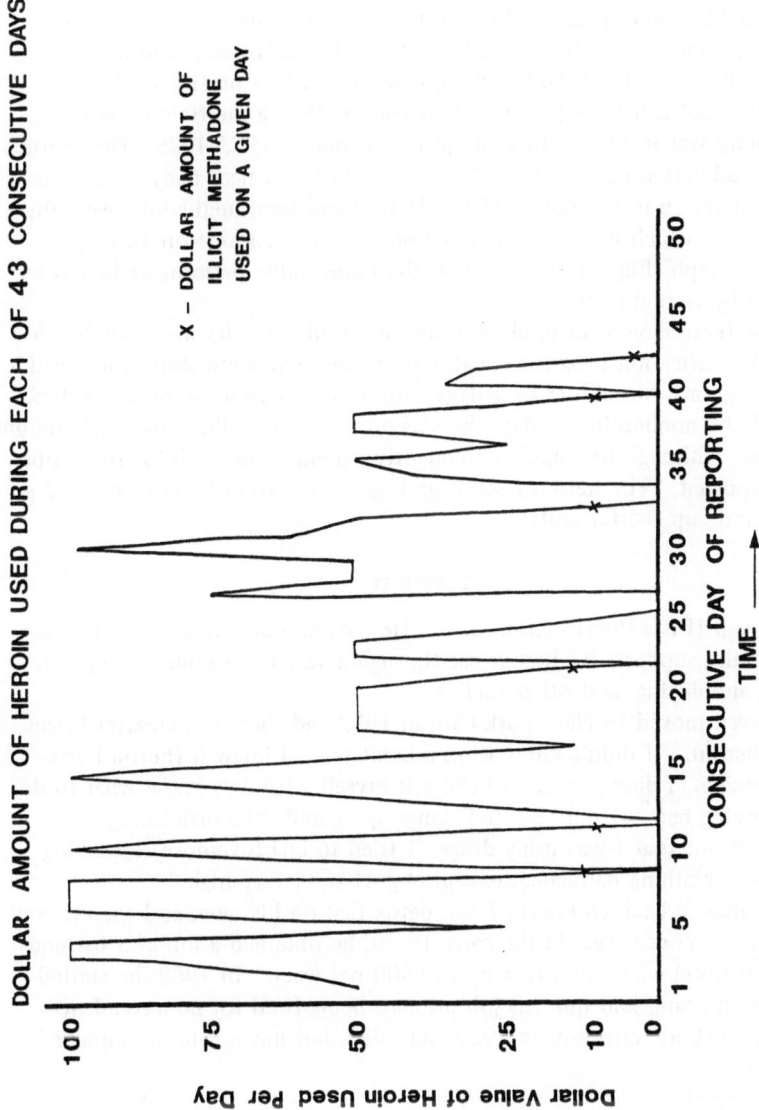

Fig. 1. Daily heroin use of Theo W.

While he has committed many different offenses (burglary, robbery, purse snatching, mugging, shoplifting), he was mainly involved in dealing heroin. A house connection gives him 25 "dime" ($10) bags and he must return back $175. Thus, he has the potential of a $75 profit; but he must frequently "sell short" (sell several bags for less than a multiple of 10).

Sonny was in two methadone programs during 1973-1979. He returned to heroin addiction immediately afterwords and was a near daily heroin user when interviewed in the fall of 1979. Heroin and legal methadone were the only drugs to which he reported addiction. He uses cocaine on an irregular basis. His graph (Fig. 2) shows one of the more stable patterns of heroin use exhibited by respondents.

The three days with nonheroin use occurred while he was attending a 14-day detoxification program (small circles represent methadone consumed at this program), but so did four days with $50 of heroin use between these. On all of the nonheroin use days, he was on the street selling his usual amount of heroin. Although his supplier frequently supplied him with "heroin" tips, Sonny reported, "The heroin I sell is garbage. I sell what he gives me and go uptown and cop (better stuff)."

Steven H

Steven H is a Puerto Rican male. He uses heroin several times per day and generally supports his heroin use through a variety of crimes (burglary, robbery, shoplifting, and other thefts).

Steven moved to New York City in 1959 and shortly thereafter began sniffing heroin. "I didn't know what a habit was. I knew it (heroin) was habit forming. I didn't want to believe it myself. I didn't know what to do. I kept buying bags. Then I started skinpopping and then mainlining. My wife found out that I was using drugs. I tried to OD (overdose) by taking three bags. Nothing happened, except (I got) very, very high."

He moved back to Puerto Rico, detoxified on his own, and then moved back to New York City. In the early 1960s, he obtained a job as a bartendar at a major hotel where he made up to $500 per week. In 1968, he started using heroin again, and quit his job prior to being fired for nonattendance. He had two short term jobs in 1969 and 1970, but has not been employed since then.

During the 1970s, he supported himself by shoplifting, robbery, burglary, and theft from cars, but has never been involved in pimping, con games, dealing, or gambling. "I am a loner. Do you see me with someone? I like to be by myself."

In 1970 Steven reported, ". . . There wasn't any (methadone) programs like now anywhere. I went to this doctor on West Street. (The doctor gave me) pills; they used to give me seven biscuits (dolophine tablets) a week for

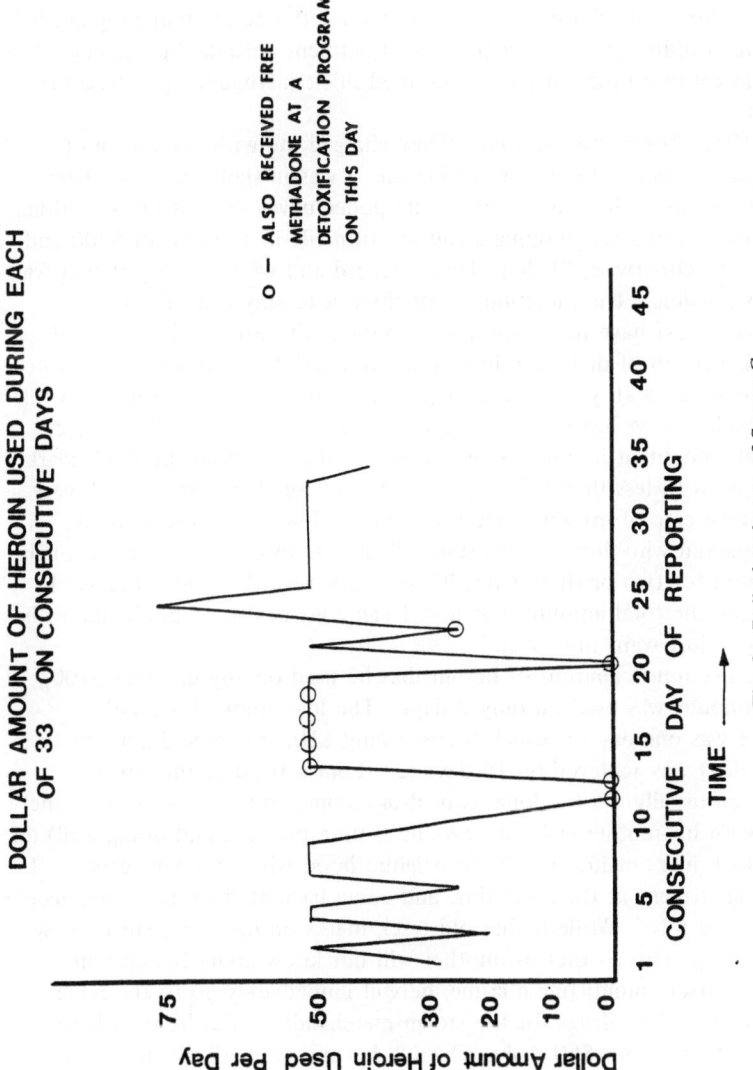

Fig. 2. Daily heroin use of Sonny C.

$20. It was only for two months, because they closed the place; they was doing something out of order. They gave me a letter to another program if I wanted to. I didn't go." Other than this treatment episode, he has never been enrolled in another program nor has he used illicit methadone purchased from the street.

In 1972 Steven was arrested, "They charged me with possession of a hypodermic needle, and two bags of heroin. I was in (jail) 18 days. They dismissed the case, I have no record. The police never showed up or nothing." He was also arrested for jumping a subway turnstile in 1978 (with $200 and two tokens). Otherwise, "I don't have a record and want to keep it that way as long as possible. The most important thing is to stay out of jail."

Project staff have now maintained contact with Steven H for over three years. His pattern of daily heroin consumption exhibited during the first 46 days has continued all year. His average consumption is about $50 and while quite variable, shows less daily variation (Fig. 3) than several other subjects. "My usual amount of heroin is one "quarter" (about $50 on the illicit market). I can get by with less than half a quarter ($25). But I seldom get sick very often. I take care of myself." He is one of the few heroin users among those contacted who does not consume all that he buys. "If I make enough, I buy heroin for two or three days, it's less expensive that way. Before, I used to take the total amount, but now I can control this. I don't like to be very high. I just want my usual."

The maximum amount of heroin that he used on any day was $100, but this amount was used on only 2 days. The low point of Steven's heroin use was one day on which he used only $10. His modal amount ($50 per day) was achieved on 16 days (or about a third of the days).

Steven usually works alone, cops drugs alone, and uses his drugs alone. He lives with his mother (who believes he is on a program and doing well) on a good block just outside the ghetto neighborhood where he cops drugs. "I leave my apartment at the same time and come back at the same time; people think I have a job." While he has old track marks on his arms, Steven now injects into leg veins so that his mother will not know about his current addiction. After committing a crime, he will immediately go to the same dealer who gives him drugs for the stolen merchandise. But he used heroin on every day, at about $50 daily. Overall, his appearance is so neat that he has had trouble buying drugs because dealers suspect him of being an undercover policeman. He never loiters with other heroin users on street corners and seldom visits with heroin-using friends.

In many ways, Steven controls his daily heroin consumption, presents himself as a respectable working person, avoids contact with other addicts, and successfully conceals his current heroin use from his mother and neighbors. Thus, he is seldom labeled as an addict by others, although he presents considerable evidence of being currently physically dependent.

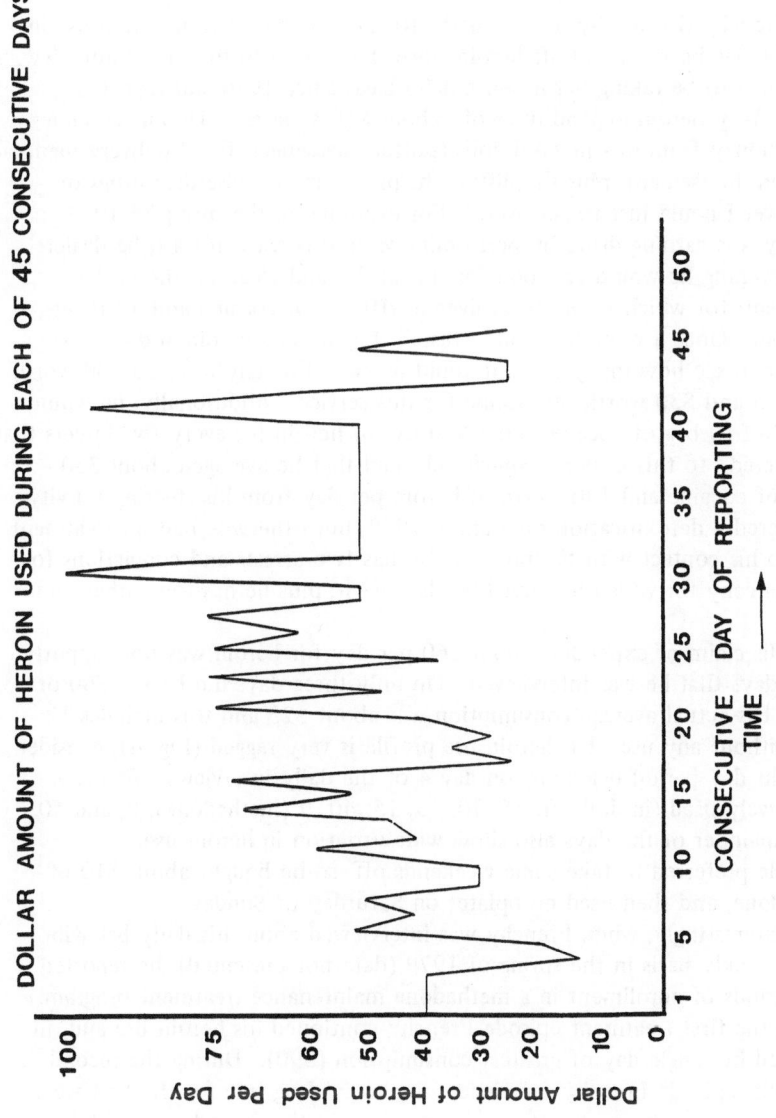

Fig. 3. Daily heroin use of Steven H.

Frenchy S

Frenchy S is a 33-year-old Puerto Rican male who began heroin use in 1963; he has been on and off heroin since that time. In the initial interview, he claimed to be taking heroin on a daily basis since 1976 and reported current daily heroin expenditures of "about $60 at least." He makes some of his money from off-the-book jobs (porter, messenger, floral delivery man, doorman, houseman), plus shoplifting, helping someone else deal drugs or "whatever I could just to get over." For example, in the spring of 1979 Frenchy was earning drugs by performing various services for a drug dealer. Every evening he would get food for this dealer and clean up the dealer's apartment, for which Frenchy received a $10 bag of cocaine and a $10 bag of heroin. Once a week he would "taste" this dealer's heroin and cocaine in order to see how many times it could be cut. Frenchy received $30 worth of heroin and $30 worth of cocaine for this service. Additionally, he would receive a $10 bag of cocaine and a $10 bag of heroin for every five buyers that he "steered" to this dealer. Frenchy claimed that he averaged about $30 worth of cocaine and $30 worth of heroin per day from his steering activity. He entered a detoxification program in 1978, but otherwise had no treatment prior to his contact with the project. He has two arrests and convictions for grand larceny for which he served 90 days each; plus he has four other minor arrests.

His claim of expending about $60 per day for heroin was not supported in the days that he was interviewed. On only three days did he use $60 or more. His actual average consumption was about $25 and this includes 12 days without any use. His heroin use profile is very ragged (Fig. 4); consider the eight day period beginning on day 4 of the daily interviews. Frenchy successively used (in dollars): 15, 70, 35, 15, 40, 9 (methadone), 0, and 50. The remainder of the days also show wide variation in heroin use.

He preferred to take some weekends off, so he bought about $10 of methadone, and then used no opiates on Saturday or Sunday.

Interestingly, when Frenchy was interviewed about his daily behavior over a weekly basis in the spring of 1979 (data not presented), he reported two periods of enrollment in a methadone maintenance treatment program. During the first treatment episode Frenchy continued his heroin use and, in fact, had his single day of greatest consumption ($90). During the second treatment episode Frenchy remained completely drug free for the first week but returned to his usual pattern of heroin use in the second week, while receiving licit methadone.

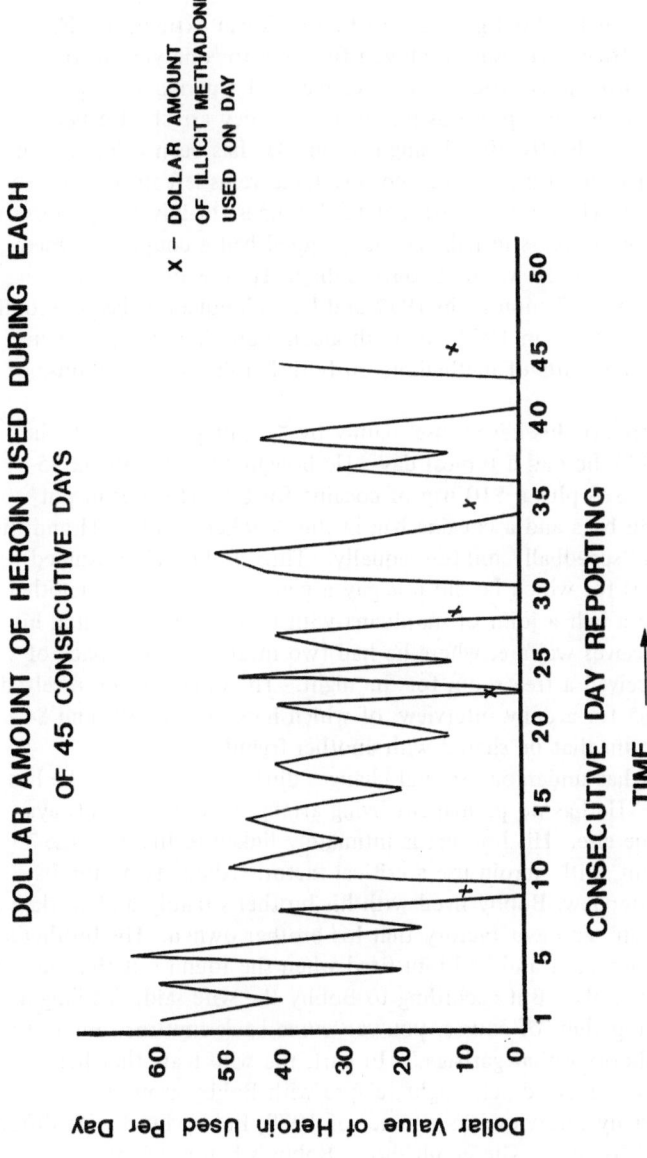

Fig. 4. Daily heroin use of Frenchy S.

Bobby H

Bobby H is a high school graduate of Puerto Rican extraction. His father is a police officer. He was employed full-time for one year in the early 1960s as a corrections officer but never received a permanent appointment, probably because of a previous minor delinquency arrest. He began using heroin in 1965, shortly after losing his job. He has been using heroin quite regularly since that time and has no injectable veins left in his arm, so he injects in his leg. He has been arrested 12–14 times (mainly for possession), and has served about 6 years in jail. He has jumped bail a couple of times and currently has two arrest warrants outstanding. He was on a private methadone program for 3 months in 1972 and has subsequently been detoxified three times, most recently in 1977, for both alcohol and heroin dependence. He also uses small amounts of methadone on both heroin use and nonuse days (Fig. 5).

Bobby H supports his heroin use mainly by "copping." Towards the end of August 1978, he had a typical day. He bought for a friend six $5 bags of heroin for $28 plus a $10 bag of cocaine for $9. This friend put three of the heroin bags and a cocaine bag in the "cooker"; Bobby H and the friend shared this "speedball" mixture equally. Thus, Bobby H consumed about $12 of drugs for which he did not pay a penny. He also met another friend who shared a half a joint of marijuana with him. Then he visited his girlfriend, who receives welfare, where he had two meals, used her pack of cigarettes, and received a free room for the night. The only cash he received on this day was $5 for a daily interview, of which he gave his girlfriend $4 and spent $1 on rum that he shared with another friend.

Bobby's life has undergone several changes during the year that he has been interviewed. He has no permanent living arrangement but has always lived with someone else. His housing is intimately linked to his drug use and/or employment, with heroin use a critical factor. About two months before the first interview, Bobby lived with his brother's family and worked at a small "sweat shop" garment factory that his brother owned. His brother's wife had Bobby move out and had him fired when she found out that he was using heroin too heavily. But according to Bobby the wife said, "as long as you get yourself together, of course, you can come back anytime, but I just don't want you shooting that garbage." In part, the wife fears that her husband, who is a former addict, might relapse with Bobby around.

During his daily interviews in summer of 1978, Bobby lived with different persons, mainly girlfriends. The graph shows Bobby's heroin use was consistently low. Of the 71 days for which data were collected, he used $50 worth of heroin once, $40 twice, and $30 or less the remainder of the time. On 14 of the 71 days (20%) he used no heroin at all, although he used illicit methadone. He claimed a $25 per day habit but during the summer of 1978

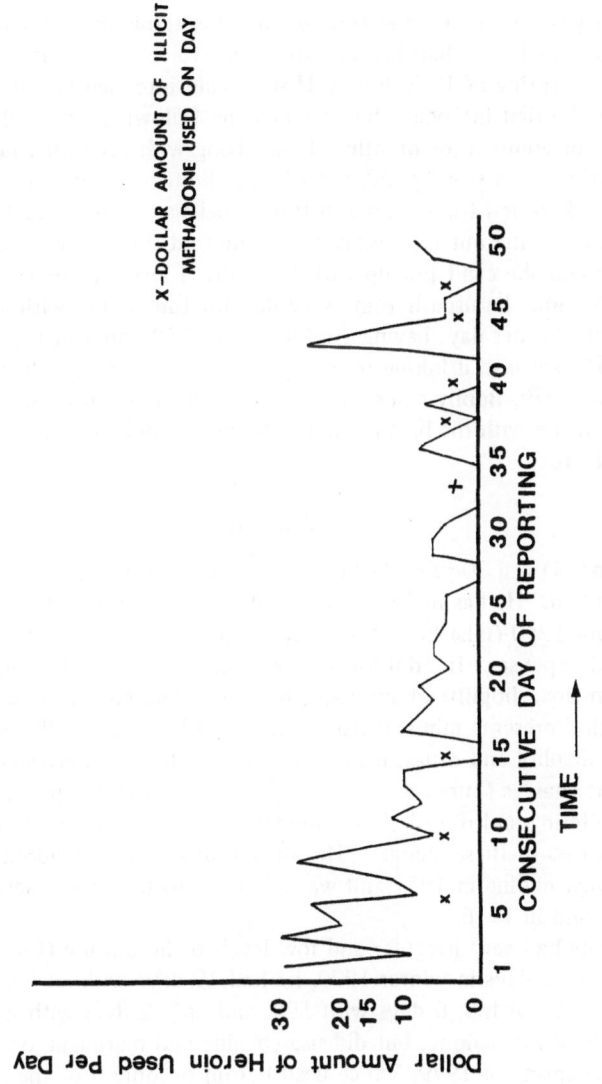

Fig. 5. Daily heroin use of Bobby H.

(daily interviews), averaged only about $9. Most of this heroin was received as drug payments for steering and copping; his actual cash expenditures for drugs were much less than his use (Johnson, Goldstein, and Preble, 1979).

In the spring of 1979 Bobby H was again interviewed but on a weekly basis. At the first interview, he provided the following story: "I was doing beautiful for about three months. I was living with my girlfriend, really doing good, working as a stone grinder—$3.10 per hour with overtime, cleared $190 per week. I started fooling around three weeks ago dibbing and dabbing. The girl kicked me out two weeks ago. She said she has two growing daughters and she can't put up with this shit. I lost my job a week ago." During the time, he used heroin every day for four weeks with a mean amount of $22 per day, having a minimum of $12 and a high of $50 of heroin. He was also drinking over a quart of wine per day. In the late summer of 1979, Bobby's heroin use had declined and became irregular. He was back living with his brother and sister-in-law and working at the brother's clothing factory.

Vance D

Vance D is a 30-year-old black who lives with a common law wife and three children. He has had a full-time job since 1969 in a florist shop. He earns about $250 (take home) per week and gives $225 to his wife for household expenses. In addition to the remaining $25 of his salary, he earns $40–50 in tips, shoplifts about twice per week, and engages in a burglary when the occasion presents minimal risk of arrest. Almost all of this money is spent for alcohol and drugs, mainly heroin. He has been arrested 12–14 times on various charges (burglary, robbery, possession of stolen property, but mainly loitering and disorderly conduct); he served about 2½ years in jail or prison on two of these charges. He was enrolled in a methadone program for about a year ending in 1977 and was admitted to the prison detox unit at Riker's Island in 1976.

Vance had very irregular and low levels of heroin use (Fig. 6). During 35 consecutive days in winter 1979, he had 19 days without heroin use, 8 days using $10 or less, 6 days with $20, and only 2 days with more. He used no illicit methadone, but did use cocaine and marijuana on occasion. During the spring of 1979, Vance used heroin on only 5 of the 28 days for which he was interviewed. He consumed $50 worth of heroin on one occasion, $25 on two occasions, $10 once and $15 once.

In the spring of 1979 Vance had lost about 50 pounds, apparently due to increased alcohol consumption (now over a quart of wine per day). He also used heroin ($35) on two separate occasions during a typical week. His heroin use has remained sporadic, but his alcohol dependence has grown and is negatively affecting his health.

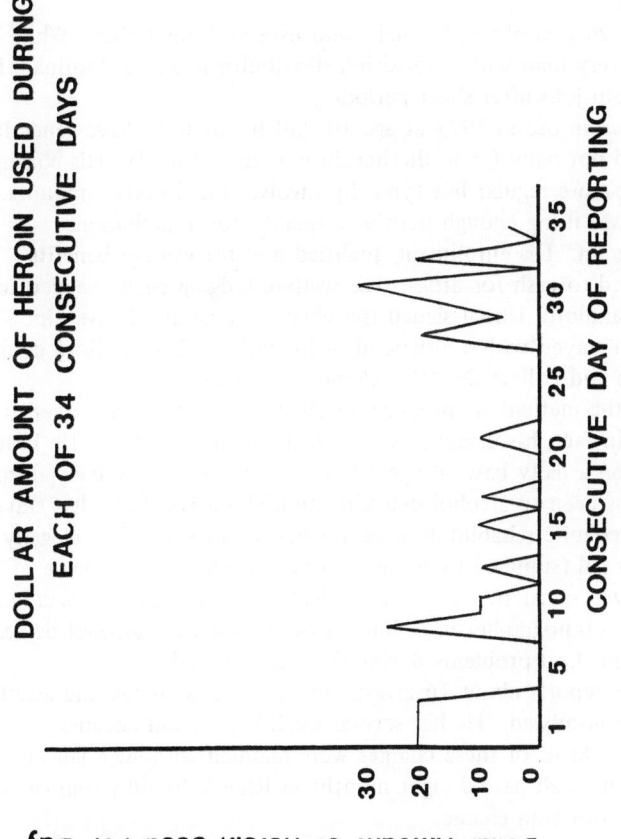

Fig. 6. Daily heroin use of Vance D.

Ulric Q

Ulric Q is a 24-year-old white male who lives with his father. While he had jobs as a delivery man with a softdrink distributor and as a doorman, he was fired from both jobs after short periods.

He began heroin use in 1971 at age 14, but his patterns have generally been irregular and not daily (as in the heroin use chart, Fig. 7). His consumption of cocaine is more regular but typically involves small dollar amounts. Nevertheless, he was using enough heroin to qualify for a methadone maintenance program. His enrollment qualified him for welfare benefits which he converted to cash for drugs. His welfare lodging check needed to be cosigned by the landlord; Ulrich signed the check, the landlord gave him $25 to $30 and Ulrich stayed with a girlfriend or his father. The landlord could rent out his room and collect the $96 payment from welfare.

He was on the methadone program in 1975–76 but was discharged for heavy drinking. In fact, his drinking has been the major problem. He began drinking alcohol on a daily basis at age 12 and has been a heavy daily drinker ever since. He has been to alcohol detoxification about six times, has stayed at a temporary alcoholic rehabilitation center many times, and has illegally bought alcohol in jail (supplied by a jail employee). During the course of this research, he was constantly in such an alcoholic stupor that he was hard to interview. The ethnographer took him to the hospital for alcohol detoxification and other medical problems during the study period.

Although he reports about 16 arrests, including a homicide and assault charge, both were dismissed. He has several small heroin and cocaine possession charges. Most of these charges were handled without a jail or prison sentence, although he did eight months in Riker's Island jail in early 1978 for a parole violation charge.

He is a low-level hustler, doing almost anything except major crime to gain a dollar. Most of his hustles are very low level. Steering, touting, and copping drugs are very common. The following transaction is typical. A friend may say, "I got ten pills to sell for $6." Later Ulric meets a person who wants to buy the pills. Ulric charges $8 for the 10 pills making two dollars, "plus the guy I bought it for will give me $1–$2 and the juy I sold it for, he'll give me $1 or $2." Thus, he may make $4–$6 off the transaction. He also sells loose joints (marijuana) and does odd jobs. His daily income is low and so is his drug use.

DISCUSSION

These case histories only touch upon the fascinating patterns of heroin use which influence the lives of these subjects. Several major findings emerge.

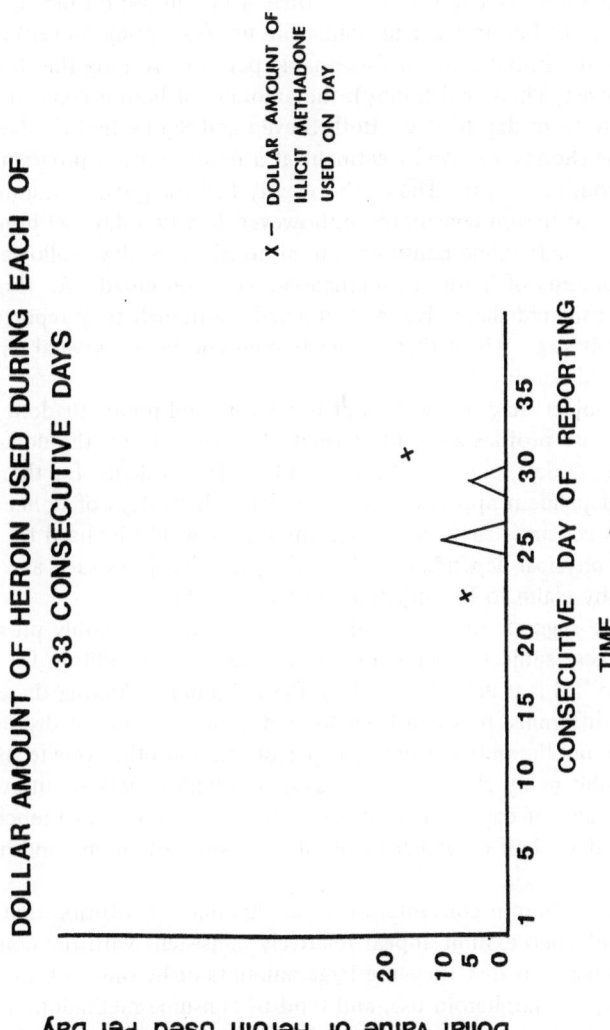

Fig. 7. Daily heroin use of Ulric Q.

All of the subjects show relatively ragged prifiles of heroin use during consecutive days. Days of heroin use and nonheroin use (excepting Steven) are typically intermixed without a major discernable pattern. Among the three heaviest users (Steven, Theo, and Sonny), the amounts of heroin consumed varied considerably from day to day. Both Steven and Sonny had no days without opiate use (Sonny received treatment at a detoxification program during his nonheroin use days). Theo, who clearly had the greatest number of days with $100 of heroin consumption, however, had two days without any heroin or illicit methadone consumption, although these days followed days when low amounts of heroin or methadone were consumed. All three of the subjects considered themselves as "addicted", although they reported having a small habit size. All of these subjects used cocaine on several days when they also used heroin.

The other subjects had many days of nonheroin and nonmethadone use. Their heroin use profiles are quite ragged. On days of use, the dollar amounts are quite modest, generally $20 or under. The evidence for their being physically dependent appears slim because they have days of nonheroin use and appear to consume such small amounts that it would be hard to demonstrate true physical dependence, although several subjects such as Frenchy and Bobby claim to be addicted and have a habit.

This evidence suggests that physical dependence, while possibly present among a few of these subjects, seems not to be a necessary condition for current "addiction" as is usually believed by the lay public. Among these heroin users, the difference between Frenchy and Sonny are one of degree. In the eyes of the public, police, treatment personnel, and other opiate users, both subjects exhibit many characteristics associated with beliefs about addiction. Yet the number of days of heroin use differ considerably, as Frenchy has many nonuse days, half of which involved illicit methadone use and half which did not.

The patterns of heroin consumption or methadone substitution that Steven, Sonny, and Theo exhibit appear relatively consistent with the concept of physical dependence in that they use large amounts of heroin on typical days, have few days of nonheroin use, and tend to consume methadone on nonheroin days. Yet if they are physically dependent, questions arise about the minimum amount they must consume to avoid withdrawal and how much they need to achieve euphoria. In addition, they state that they have small habits, if any, due to the poor quality of street heroin. Their heroin consumption may also be due to a *belief* that they are physically dependent, rather than exhibiting a true physiological state of withdrawal if they do not use the drug.

For the other subjects, especially Frenchy and Bobby, their patterns of heroin consumption appear quite regular although not daily, but the amounts are smaller, methadone substitution somewhat more common, and the means of support appear different. The regular heroin users (including Frenchy, Bobby, and Vance) use heroin on about 60 percent of the days, but typically consume half as much as the near daily heroin users (including Steven, Sonny, and Theo). For the former subjects, the existence of physical dependence is either very low or nonexistent. For the irregular heroin users (including Ulric), no evidence of physical dependence to heroin is evident; sporadic use is common.

The formulation by McAuliffe and Gordon (1980), quoted at length earlier, appears to describe many of these subjects well. While physical dependence may or may not be present, many other factors also seem to be present and confound any explanation of their status of "addict" however this illusive term is defined. That is, several subjects may seem by some arbitrary definition to be physically dependent but this may not be a necessary condition for them considering themselves as "addicts," being so considered by others as "addicts," or living a lifestyle as an "addict" evident in each respondent's story.

Clearly, Bobby and Frenchy believe themselves to be physically dependent and act upon this belief to some extent, yet their actual consumption raises questions about whether they are (since they have so many days of nonuse preceded or followed by use days) as well as their degree of physical dependence. Even Vance, whose irregular patterns of heroin consumption and many days of nonheroin&nonopiate use, suggesting a controlled heroin use pattern à la Zinberg and Harding (1979), does not appear vastly different than Bobby's. Vance's commitment to his family and job appears to be the major obstacle to developing a heroin pattern similar to Bobby or Vance. As McAuliffe and Gordon (1980, 139) note, "there are important disadvantages with equating addiction with physical dependence . . . (since this idea) encourages the seriously misleading impression . . . that the user is relatively safe as long as physical dependence is avoided." While all subjects are not clearly physically dependent, they are heavily involved in an addict lifestyle.

This paper has presented patterns of heroin consumption among seven heroin users. Similar patterns of irregular heroin use could be provided for many other subjects in the study. The empirical patterns exhibited here do not fit comfortable with existing models of "addiction." These data suggest that careful analyses of daily behavior may provide new insights from which a clearer model of opiate addiction may eventually emerge, but this model appears quite distant at present.

ACKNOWLEDGMENTS

This research was supported by the New York State Division of Substance Abuse Services, by a Public Health Services Award from the National Institute on Drug Abuse (R01-DA-01926-01-03), and by an Interagency Agreement between the National Institute on Drug Abuse (R01-DA002355) and the Law Enforcement Assistance Administration (LEAA-J-IAA-005-8), U.S. Department of Justice under the Omnibus Crime Control and Safe Streets Act of 1968, as amended.

Additional support was provided by the Interdisciplinary Research Center funded by the National Institute of Justice (80-IJ-CX-0049) and by Narcotic and Drug Research, Inc.

Points of view or opinions in this document do not necessarily represent the official position or policies of the U.S. Government or the New York State Division of Substance Abuse Services.

REFERENCES

Frank B: Current drug abuse trends in New York City. Community Correspondents Group, Drug Abuse Indicator Trends, Vol. I, Forcasting Branch, Rockville, Md.: National Institute on Drug Abuse, 1979

Frank B: Current drug abuse trends in New York City. Community Correspondents Group, Drug Abuse Indicator Trends, Vol. I, Forcasting Branch, Rockville, Md.: National Institute on Drug Abuse, 1980

Johnston LD, Bachman JG and O'Malley PM: Drugs and the Nation's High School Students: 1979 Highlights. Rockville, Md.: National Institute on Drug Abuse, 1979

McAuliffe WE and Gordon A: A test of Lindesmith's theory of addiction: The frequency of euphoria among long-term addicts. *Am J Sociol* 79:795–840, 1974

McAuliffe WE and Gordon A: Issues in testing Lindesmith's theory. *Am J Sociol* 81: 154–163, 1975

McAuliffe WE and Gordon A: Conditioning and the combination-of-effects: A comprehensive reinforcement theory of opiate addiction, 1979

McAuliffe WE and Gordon A: Reinforcement and the combination of effects: Summary of a theory of opiate addiction. In: DJ Lettieri, H Sayers and H Wallenstein (eds.), *Theories on Drug Abuse: Selected Contemporary Perspectives.* Research Monograph 30, Rockville, Md.: National Institute on Drug Abuse, pp 137–141, 1980

Miller, JD and Cisin IH: *Highlights from the National Survey on Drug Abuse.* Rockville, Md.: National Institute on Drug Abuse, 1979.

O'Donnell JA et al: *Young Men and Drugs: A Nationwide Study.* Research Monograph 5, Rockville, Md.: National Institute on Drug Abuse, 1976

Robins LN: *A Follow-Up of Vietnam Drug Users.* Washington, DC: Government Printing Office, 1973

Robins LN: *The Vietnam Drug User Returns.* Special Action Office Monographs A.2. Washington, DC: Government Printing Office, 1974

Zinberg NE: Nonaddictive opiate use. In: RL Dupont, A Goldstein and J O'Donnell (eds.), *Handbook on Drug Abuse.* Rockville, Md.: National Institute on Drug Abuse, pp 303–313, 1979
Zinberg NE and WM Harding: Control over intoxicant use: A theoretical and practical overview. *Journal of Drug Issues* 9:121–143, 1979

12

Social Stress and Drug Abuse

GEORGE SERBAN

The last two decades have brought significant social and political changes
in the structure of American society and its institutions. We have witnessed
a dramatic erosion of traditional values, family life, and particularly of what
is called the Protestant ethic's attitudes toward work. The younger generation,
brought up in an affluent society, became progressively disenchanted with the
meaning of life as conceptualized by their parents and the policies of the
government.

In the midst of the ambiguity of national purpose of the sixties and
seventies, one appealing answer was to avoid all social confrontation and to
return to the natural state of things expressed by non-involvement, detach-
ment, and search for reaching a state of happiness—even if artificially induced.
Society became progressively more hedonistically oriented and, with it, more
drug oriented. In this context, working hard became meaningless to the
young generation; stresses of life were supposed to be avoided at any price,
and the panacea for going through life was found in drugs.

Barbiturates, valium, and quaaludes became the easiest means to cope
with any discomfort of living. To understand the staggering amount of the
abuse of drugs, in 1978, 280 million prescriptions for psychoactive drugs had
been written according to the last report of HEW; 13 million Americans have
used stimulants without medical supervision; 9.3 million are using sedatives;
and 7.8 million are taking tranquilizers. According to DAWN (Drug Abuse
Warning Network), between January and December of 1978, 117,023 drug
consultations took place in emergency rooms related to drug abuse. The use
of drugs to induce peace of mind became a way of life for an important
segment of our population.

In addition, drugs were used to add a new dimension to the individual's recreational life. For instance, marijuana became considered the drug of choice for creating a relaxed state of mind which would be beneficial to the individual in stressful social or intimate situations.

Between 41 and 47 million Americans have tried marijuana, and between 16 and 20 million use it regularly. It became the prevalent substance used by older adolescents and young adults. Though it is claimed to be a "safe" drug, medical research proved to the contrary. The same applies to PCP (angel dust) which is used by approximately 14 percent of the young adult population between 18 and 25. The medical consequences of this drug are disastrous, leading to violent antisocial behavior, depression, or death.

In general, the logic behind the use of these drugs is simple. Since we live in an age of anxiety, the best way to combat it is with a drug that will numb us to unwarranted social pressures. But for some, to relax was not enough. They wanted to control their state of mind according to the need of the moment. They wanted to be stimulated beyond the ordinary pleasurable experiences of life. They were bored with the routine of life. They were seekers of new thresholds of excitement; otherwise, life was too depressing. For some, speed was the drug of choice; it made someone feel good, leaving all problems behind them and requiring no further solution. It is estimated that about four million Americans have received in 1977 prescriptions for amphetamines, and about 1.8 million obtained them illicitly. Some of them were indirectly acquired under the guise of appetite supressants. In addition, they are used under the belief that it changes the personality and makes the person feel more desirable socially, more entertaining, more "in control" of situations.

The ill effects of these drugs are too well known to be discussed. Not to mention that after getting high someone addicted in order "to come down" or to go to sleep has to use barbiturates. The ups and downs become another modality to cope with life, giving people the illusion of living life with high intensity while, in reality, they slowly disorganize their lives to the point of removing themselves from the mainstream of social life.

If this is part of the scene of the colleges and of the middle class, where people still pretend to be integrated into the fabric of society, for some people from the lower social economic class apparently the situation is somewhat different. They go for the real stuff; they get high with heroin. We have approximately 600,000 hard core addicted to heroin; now, with the latest heroin epidemic, their number might increase as well.

There are many social and economic reasons to explain why heroin infiltrated so deeply into the lower social economic class while marijuana and soft tranquilizers appealed to the middle class and cocaine became the drug of choice of the upper class. One of the reasons was the system of distribution of heroin which was done through the lower social economic class. The spread of heroin was in spurts and at times became epidemic according to the availability of the drug and the activity of the pushers (Feldman, 1968). Regardless of the drug of choice of the social class, it could be safely assumed at this point that the spread of drugs could be attributed to the social sickness of our society, where the norms of conduct and expectations from individuals are broken down; where its permissiveness and tolerance to crime produced by drug addiction encouraged further the abuse of drugs.

In this context we can say that the motives for taking drugs and starting a career as a drug abuser, as have already been described in literature, are related to thrill seeking, curiosity, relaxation, sense of well being, instant gratification and peer acceptance, yet they do not explain why the drug user becomes addicted. Why does one become dependent on the drug instead of taking it only occasionally, for instance, in socially entertaining situations? Though most of potential drug users are introduced to it by a trusted friend who wants to share with him the experience of getting high, it does not tell us why some will continue on drugs and others will not. The argument that the addict becomes addicted because of his friends does not hold under closer scrutiny. Not everyone will stay a junkie in order to maintain the friendship and get the approval of his friends who are taking it.

Although, admittedly, drug novice is initiated in the drug activity sometimes ignorant of the long term effect of the drug but, persuaded by his friends of its favorable effects, it does not explain why he continues after seeing the ill effects of it.

One scientific explanation for addiction is based on the assumption that the individual is unable to give up the drug because of the unpleasant effects of withdrawal. In fact, the classical theory of drug addiction was based on the concept of Lindesmith that the chronic drug abuser does not get high any more on the drug, but is forced to use it in order to feel "normal", free of withdrawal's signs (McAuliffe, 1974). Though this might be partially true, it does not explain why drug addicts, after successfully withdrawing from a drug, later go back to it repeatedly. It is well known that approximately 70 percent of drug addicts return to drugs within two years after their abstinence (Fracchia, 1976). It means that the element of pleasure which he experienced by taking the drug is still the main motivating factor in resuming the habit.

This is supported by the conclusion of McAuliffe and others who found that the drug dependent person continues to use the drug not only because of fear of withdrawal but because he wants to get high in at least 40 percent of the cases (Serban, 1978). In these terms, the drug abuser does not take drugs to ward off the unpleasantness of withdrawal but because he created his own world of living in which the reality of his life, perceived as unpleasant, is replaced with a continuous state of pleasure induced by the use of drugs.

These two theoretical hypotheses have serious social and psychological implications. If the basic assumption of Lindesmith's theory that the drug dependent abuses the drug in the need to avoid the suffering of withdrawal, then obviously the successful withdrawal from the drug should cure the disease. But, on the other hand, if the drug addict is a pleasure seeker with a low motivation for integration into society, even after he is successfully freed from the drug he still poses serious problems in terms of the ability to successfully cure him.

These theoretical models and these different conceptualizations of the etiology of drug addiction are reflected in the diversity of therapeutic approaches. The whole concept of heroin substitutes like methadone, LAAM, etc, is based on the assumption that the established addiction is hard to change and as such should be maintained by more controlled means of the same drug, or at best to reduce its use by a slow process leading, whenever possible, to the discontinuation of the drug. In this context, other approaches like that of easing of withdrawal signs by the use of clonidine or lofexidine will work out in the long term provided that the individual is not attempting to reexperience the initial "rush," the feeling of high. Otherwise, the withdrawal is useless since this need will bring him back to taking the drug whenever past psycho-social difficulties created by the drug will be forgotten. Even the use of a "perfect" drug such as naltrexone, which suppresses the euphoric effect of heroin, is of no value if the addict refuses to take it because he voluntarily wants to feel high.

In reality, it is a fact that most hard-core drug addicts enroll in the program when they have serious brushes with the law and are unable to support their habit anymore. This is why the social rehabilitation process starts only when the addict has reached his lowest physical, emotional and social point in order to make him feel that any available social alternative of support is salutory. These specific factors add new dimensions to the problem of drug addiction, making it more elusive to cure regardless of the implementation of various medical treatments or social rehabilitation programs.

For all these reasons, another closer look might be necessary to be taken to approach this multidimensional problem. It appears that a constellation of factors are significant in the orientation of the initial drug taker toward a career of a lifetime of abuse. In the forefront of the constellation is his orientation toward immediate gratification combined with an inability to cope with the problems of his life and a magical organization of thinking, they appear to be necessary for the beginning of the drug abuse career. This particular cognitive—emotional approach to events of life and to frustration with the social environment leads the individual to experience lack of success in reaching his goals. It results later on in an underlying depression and a sense of futility due to his inability to meet his expectations. However, the magical elements of his thinking, where he believes he is able to withdraw from the drug as he pleases because he is in control of himself, contribute to the experimentation with drugs. This attitude, superimposed on the need to look for immediate, painless solutions to his life problem, reinforces his addiction. In general, the problems of the addict could be reduced to a particular mode of viewing life in which a permissive and conducive social environment acts as a reinforcer.

The assumption made by some clinicians about the existence of an addictive personality is in reality a post hoc, after effect description of the state of addiction. Many characteristics have been attributed to the addict personality. Obviously, the first one is that of obsessive compulsive behavior about the use of drugs. But this is a circular explanation. Other researchers found out that addicts have a tendency to equate needs for success and independence with nonconformity and experimentation. They have difficulty in interpersonal relationships, inability to have friends and intrapsychic conflicts revolving around dependency (Lawrence, 1973). All might be true, but still this cannot explain the addiction as based on a simple need for acceptance and socialization where in long term the contrary is true. He becomes more alienated from community and friends.

The second controversial issue is the contribution of a depressive personality or a depressive condition to the use of drugs. In our own research, confirmed by others, we have found a strong depressive component favoring the habituation to drugs. In fact, in a pilot study done at NYU in which we have treated 117 ex-methadone and soft drug addicts with only antidepressants and anxiolytics, we found that 54 percent of soft drug abusers became abstinent for a period of nine months followup. In this group, particularly for some ex-methadone, depression appeared to be the main factor for continuation of drug abuse, but not for beginning its use. However, for the soft drug addict, the need for psychoactive or stimulant drugs was due mainly to inability to cope with stresses of life which led to frustration and experimentation with drugs (1981).

The need to get high, to feel relaxed, might be related in some drug addicts to the underlying depression possibly intensified by the disturbance in the pleasure centers induced by heroin (Hunt, 1971). The role of endorphin in the development and maintenance of addiction is not yet fully elucidated.

Though it is common knowledge for the drug abusers to switch easily from one category of drug abuse to another, sometimes combining both, the fact remains that the hard core drug addict finds it extremely difficult to give up his heroin need or to switch to a soft drug even after the physiological dependence has been eliminated.

Yet all these personality aspects cannot explain the etiology of drug addiction since some hard core addicts are able to remain abstinent while others are not. It means that other psychological and social factors are contributing to the maintenance of addiction which appear to be related to the style and concept of life of the addicted, as previously mentioned. Due to these factors, the taking of the drug, after the initial curiosity or need for thrill seeking, becomes a necessity and a habit. For him, it represents not only a solution to a gamut of unsolved conflicts with which he's unable to cope, but it reaches a state of emotional comfort unable to give up. The initial feelings of getting high and the desire for "the rush" stay with him and he craves to relive it again and again as a compensation for his underlying *perceived* meaninglessness of life.

This is true too to some extent for the soft drug abuser. It is self-evident that the marijuana or stimulant user is psychologically addicted to maintaining a state of pleasure against the adversities of life. In the same context, we may find an explanation for the recent fad of cocaine use. Successful people from the world of art, movies and television are using it to enhance their sense of well being beyond the point of the natural experience of pleasure to a state of euphoria.

The need for a pleasurable state of mind sought by cocaine users could be translated in the illegal import of approximately 66 thousand pounds, totalling an expenditure of around 20 billion dollars a year (1981). Basically, there is not too much difference between the Harlem addicted and the Hollywood–New York entertainers who, in the final analysis, are taking drugs, be it heroin or cocaine, to transcend whatever they perceive as painful or unpleasant in their lives, or to attempt to reach the final state of ataraxia—peace of mind. Both groups may start for similar reasons; either sheer curiosity or peer acceptance, of sharing the experience of getting high, be it in a dark alley between the dilapidated buildings of Harlem or in a sumptuous living room of a Beverly Hills–Park Ave. mansion. Both groups want to push the threshold of the reality, defined as unpleasant for the Harlem people and boring unstimulating for Hollywood–New York, into the realm of euphoria.

The nagging question to be asked is why this need for drug addicts to maintain a constant state of happiness when life presupposes an amount of unpleasant, effortful processes? Is it because they are mentally ill? Apparently, here starts the confusion between the medical model and the social model utilized to understand addicts.

The medical model supports the hypothesis that drug addiction is a metabolic illness comparable to that of diabetes, an analogy liked by the exponents of this hypothesis. It is assumed that the metabolic disturbance produced by the long term use of heroin is due to the interference with normal release of various types of endorphin into the central nervous system. As a result, the addict has a psychophysiological imbalance, translated into a disturbance in equilibrium of the pleasure centers resulting in a craving for heroin. Though there is some evidence to partially favor this hypothesis, still it does not explain why some drug addicts are able to become abstinent while others are not. Based on this concept, the attempt to cure drug addiction is futile, and the only solution will be long-term maintenance on heroin, methadone, LAAM.

The opponents of this concept believe drug addiction is a pure social problem, a modality of coping with the environment, an attitude toward life that is a search for pleasure. In this context, after the initial period of withdrawal, the individual has a choice to stay sober, abstinent or not.

While it's true that the medical model did not come up with the final answer to the etiology of drug addiction and might have confounded some pathogenic conditions produced by it with its etiology, in other words, the effect with the cause, yet there is enough evidence that psychophysiological factors are heavily involved in the maintenance of addiction.

By the same token, the social factors reinforcing and maintaining the addiction cannot be overlooked. Their totality is responsible for making the addict a career pleasure seeker. In this context, drug addiction appears to be a bio-psychosocial disease in which both sets of factors are reinforcing each other negatively in maintaining the condition. It means that the detoxification must be a medical problem but not necessarily the only problem of addiction. The value of the medical model necessarily stops here unless the patient is placed on a maintenance program such as methadone or LAAM. The over-looking of the psychosocial aspects of the problems of addiction and the specific personality responses explains the limited success with drug abusers either in treating or preventing their relapses.

The disregard for the social mode might explain why most of the drug addicts are unwilling to follow any course of treatment. Not to mention that the use of one treatment for one category of patients is totally unsuccessful for another group. This heterogeneity of causes producing addiction appears to be responsible for the wide spectrum of treatment, claiming success with such diverse and contradictory approaches.

Finally, the common denominator which should be sought by all this treatment, after the individual is detoxified by medication or without it in a "cold turkey" fashion, is to change his state of mind, for acceptance of the unpleasant reality of life with the accompanying daily problems which he has to face and solve. On the other hand, it is nothing new about this need of the individual to transcend reality. Since time immemorial, man has attempted to transcend the unpleasant reality by escaping in reverie, meditation or artificial use of herbs and seeds with sedative or hallucinogenic effects. Now, a new dimension has been added to it.

Our society is strongly committed to the utopian goal of elimination of pain, suffering and discomfort. The drug addict appears to be "the avant-garde" of these new aims; they are the forerunners in the pursuit of happiness. Let us not forget that happiness is a human invention, as St. Just remarked during the French Revolution; its pursuit does indeed require artificial means of reaching and experiencing.

Finally, what role does stress play in the extensive use of drugs? It is a fact that the more complicated society becomes, the more stresses it induces in its citizens and the less people are able to cope with it, which means that they might experience more anxiety and/or depression. In a recent study at NYU investigating the amount of stress experienced by the population between 18 and 60 in the United States, we have found that approximately 70 percent of the population is under moderate to heavy stress. The stress is produced by the rapid social changes affecting the interaction and the role of the sexes, marital relationships, the job and other economic hardships. People who cannot cope with these stresses were found to rely on religion, sometimes magic and others on drugs. It should also be mentioned that 51.9 percent of the men and 60.1 percent of the women experience high to moderate anxiety, while 34.2 percent of the men and 41.3 percent of the women experience depressive episodes (Serban, 1981). The staggering use of valium and alcohol in our society is said to be related to stress.

It is assumed that nine million people are alcohol abusers and 200,000 deaths yearly that are related to alcohol seem due to the stress of life. It is said that the more stressful the human interaction becomes, the more increase we will see in the use of alcohol or drugs; up to a point this is true. According to some statistics, in the past 15 years alcohol consumption increased about 30 percent. In addition, 90 million prescriptions for only minor tranquilizers were filled, according to the statistics of 1977. Yet, these data convey, at best, a meaningful connection between stress and drug abuse; we cannot say that the large proportion of alcohol abusers attempt to control stress in their overindulgence in alcohol. Basically, more of them regardless of stress are closer to the group of pleasure seekers—the drug users.

If stress plays a minor role in the alcoholic addiction—it plays even less of one in the abuse of drugs by teenagers.

The four million adolescents between 12 and 17 who are using marijuana and the 1.5 million who use PCP are using it for pleasure and not because of the stress in their lives. And the same applies to 8.5 million marijuana and 4.2 million PCP users between 17 and 25. It is estimated that about 37 percent of the high school students use marijuana periodically, and 11 percent of them are using it daily as recreational.

It is a mistake to assume that most of the soft drug users are relying on drugs to alleviate the stresses of their lives. Though some of them might start to take a sedative or mild tranquilizers in response to the stresses of life, most of them are continuing to take the drug to induce an artificial state of pleasure. This distinction is important to make because these two groups are responding differently to treatment. While the drug user who takes drugs to relieve the pressure of life could be easily treated the other one is not. The same applies to the use of drugs in the adult population. In general, the reason for the abuse of drugs by teenagers is basically that of thrill, while for adults this is not necessarily so.

It could be a combination of social and psychological reasons. In the first case the problem of relapse will not be solved unless the addicted person is ready to change his style of life, his concept of sought happiness, while in the second situation it requires also a social rehabilitation to reduce the stresses of life.

Due to the complexity of the problems involved in drug abuse, encompassing psychological, sociological, not to mention the biological aspect of it, the prevention is not necessarily successful, as proven by research, by the simple presentation to the public of the unfavorable consequences of drug use. This approach is not a deterrant for the use of drugs in a hedonistically oriented society. It requires, as well, a change in the attitude of people, a reorientation of life toward work, and toward facing and coping with the inherent adversities of life. Only in this context will the rehabilitation program be able to help the individual to develop psychological and social coping mechanisms to assess and respond realistically to life's events.

REFERENCES

Blumer H, Sutter A et al: In: Coombs R, Fry L and Lewis P (eds.) *Recruitment into Drug Use, in Socialization in Drug Abuse.* Cambridge, Mass.: Schenkman Publishing Co., 1976

Cocaine: The lethal status symbol. *MD Magazine* 25, 27:56–65, 1981

Feldman WH: Ideological supports to becoming and remaining a heroin addict. *Journal of Health and Social Behavior* 9:131–139, 1968

Fracchia J and Sheppard C: Needs of society and heroin addicts: Some general and specific implications for treatment. *Psychiatry Digest* 14–22:July, 1976

HEW: *Drug Abuse, Prevention, Treatment and Rehabilitation.* Second Annual Report, 1979

Hunt W, Barnet CW and Branch LC: Relapse rate in addiction programs. *Journal of Consulting Clinical Psychology* 4:445, 1971

Lawrence S: *Cingulate Self Stimulation in the Rat; Influence of Repeated Morphine Administration.* Proceedings, 80th Annual Convention, APA, pp 835–836, 1973

McAuliffe W and Gordon AR: A test of Lindesmith's theory of addiction: The frequency of euphoria among long term addicts. *Am J Sociol* 79(4):795–840, 1974

Serban G: New approach to the rehabilitation of the hard core drug addict (heroin methadone addicts); A pilot study. *Journal of Clinical Psychiatry* 111–116:Feb., 1978

Serban G: Present social values as possible stressors—A survey of the U.S. population. *Journal of Preventive Psychiatry* (in press)

13

Psychiatric Disorders in Treated Opiate Addicts

BRUCE J. ROUNSAVILLE
MYRNA M. WEISSMAN
HERBERT D. KLEBER
CHARLES H. WILBER

The association between opiate addiction and psychopathology has a long history which is now partially supported by empirical data. For example, opiate addicts have been shown to have high rates of depression (Dorus, 1980; Lehman, 1972; Robins, 1974; Rounsaville, 1979; Steer, 1980; Wieland, 1970; Weisman, 1976), antisocial personality characteristics (Craig, 1979), schizophrenia or schizotypal features (Sheppard, 1969; Hekimian, 1968; Zimmering, 1952), manic symptomatology (Craig, 1979; Flemmenbaum, 1974), and alcoholism (Belenko, 1979). The major problem to date, in the studies of psychopathology in opiate addicts, is the measure of psychopathology which has usually been dimensional symptom or personality scales. Diagnostic techniques, particularly the more recently improved measures, have rarely been applied to the opiate addict (Ling, 1973). The result is that there has been a gap between general psychiatric practice and the treatment of opiate abusers. This gap is reflected in the fact that opiate addicts are usually treated in separate specialty clinics. The isolation of the addict in separate treatment programs and from recent developments in psychiatric diagnostic practice could lead to missed opportunities for useful treatment. For example, the opiate addict who is also bipolar might benefit from lithium, or the addict who is also depressed, might benefit from treatment with a tricyclic antidepressant.

This paper presents data on the rates of specified psychiatric disorders according to Research Diagnostic Criteria (RDC) (Spitzer, 1978) derived from a survey of opiate addicts. While the population does not derive from a probability sample of a community, it does represent a large and heterogenous group of addicts from a variety of treatment services. With one exception

(Ling, 1973), this study represents the first published report of the newer approaches to psychiatric diagnosis applied to a sample of opiate addicts.

METHODS

Setting and Sample

Subjects were evaluated at the Yale University Drug Dependence Unit of the Connecticut Mental Health Center in New Haven, Connecticut. Psychiatric diagnosis was obtained on five hundred thirty-three (533) subjects who were contacted in the following manner: three hundred fifty-four (354) addicts were evaluated as they applied for treatment at the Screening and Evaluation Unit; one hundred twenty (120) subjects were members of the methadone maintenance program; and sixty (60) subjects were Hispanics who were evaluated in Spanish and were evaluated on application to treatment (n=30) or after entering a residential therapeutic community for Hispanic patients (n=30).

Subjects in all populations surveyed were paid for participating in the study and were interviewed only after informed written consent was obtained. For this study, opiate addiction was defined according to Research Diagnostic Criteria which require sustained regular use of opiates, signs of withdrawal when drug use is discontinued and indication that use of drugs has led to major changes in the individual's functioning (eg, committing criminal acts).

Diagnostic Techniques

Information for making diagnostic judgements was collected on the Schedule for Affective Disorders and Schizophrenia (SADS) (Endicott, 1978). On the basis of the information collected on the SADS, the subjects were classified on the Research Diagnostic Criteria (RDC) which are a set of operational diagnostic definitions with specific inclusion and exclusion criteria for a variety of nosologic groups (Spitzer, 1978).

Interviewers, Training Reliability

There were five raters with Masters and Bachelor-level education and previous experience in clinical psychiatry and interviewing. Under the supervision of a psychiatrist, the raters received three months of training on the SADS and RDC. In order to conduct interviews for this study, it was required that the rater complete five consecutive, conjoint interviews on which RDC diagnoses were in complete agreement with those of a more experienced rater. After training, reliability was periodically spot-checked on 6 percent of the sample and found to be excellent. Overall, 40 reliability interviews were completed in which one rater interviewed and a second rater observed. On the basis of these ratings, inter-rater agreement was very good with Kappa coefficients (Barthko, 1976) ranging from 0.72 to 1.0 in different diagnostic categories (Rounsaville, 1983).

RESULTS

Current Rates of Psychiatric Disorders

Current rates of disorders that are considered to have both current and past episodes are listed in Table 1. Depression is the most commonly diagnosed symptomatic condition as 23.8 percent of the sample were in a current episode of major depression at this evaluation. Other affective disorders, including minor depression (2.3 percent), manic disorders (0 percent), and hypomanic disorder (0.9 percent) were comparatively infrequently diagnosed, as were schizophrenia (0.2 percent) and schizoaffective disorders (1.5 percent). Only small fractions of the sample were in current episodes of panic (0.9 percent), obsessive compulsive (1.3 percent) or generalized anxiety (0.9 percent) disorders. However, a substantial minority had a current phobia (9.2 percent) or abused alcohol to a degree that met the criteria for a current episode of alcoholism (13.7 percent).

Table 1. Current Rates/100 of Psychiatric Disorders
in Opiate Addicts According to Research Diagnostic Criteria (N=533)

Current RDC Diagnosis	Percentage
Affective disorders	
Major depression	23.8
Minor depression	2.3
Manic disorder	0.0
Hypomanic disorder	0.9
Schizophrenia	0.2
Schizoaffective disorders	
(Depressed and manic)	1.5
Anxiety disorders	
Panic	0.9
Obsessive compulsive	1.3
Generalized anxiety	0.9
Phobic	9.2
Alcoholism	13.7
Other psychiatric disorder	4.7
Any current disorder	
(Including personality diagnoses)	70.3

Table 2. Lifetime Rates/100 RDC Psychiatric Diagnoses
in Opiate Addicts by Sociodemographic Characteristics (N=533)

Type of Disorder	Percentage
Affective disorders	
Major depression	53.9
Minor depression	8.4
Intermittent depression	18.8
Cyclothymic personality	3.6
Labile personality	16.5
Manic disorder	0.6
Hypomanic disorder	6.6
Bipolar 1 or 2	5.4
Any affective disorder	74.3
Schizophrenic disorders	
Schizophrenia	0.8
Schizoaffective depression	1.7
Schizoaffective manic	0.4
Anxiety disorders	
Panic	1.3
Obsessive compulsive	1.9
Generalized anxiety	5.4
Phobic	9.6
Any anxiety disorder	16.1
Alcoholism	34.5
Personality disorder	
Antisocial personality	26.5
Briquet's	0.2
Schizotypal features	8.4
Other psychiatric disorders	6.8
Any lifetime disorder	86.9

Lifetime Rates of Psychiatric Disorders

Table 2 shows that 86.9 percent of the addicts surveyed met the criteria for some psychiatric disorder exclusive of drug addiction in their lifetime.

Looking at the lifetime rates of specific disorders, the most commonly diagnosed disorders were major depression 53.9 percent, alcoholism 34.5 percent, antisocial personality 26.5 percent, intermittent depression 18.8 percent, labile personality 16.5 percent, phobic disorder 9.6 percent, schizotypal features 8.4 percent, minor depression 8.4 percent, other psychiatric disorders 6.8 percent, hypomanic disorder 6.6 percent, and generalized anxiety disorder 5.4 percent. All other disorders, including schizophrenia, schizoaffective disorders, mania, cyclothymic personality, obsessive compulsive disorder, panic disorder and Briquet's disorder were found in less than 5 percent of the sample. When affective disorders are combined, it is apparent that opiate addicts in this sample are at high risk in that 74.3 percent met the criteria for some affective disorder.

Multiple Diagnoses

RDC diagnoses are not mutually exclusive and multiple diagnoses were common in our sample. To evaluate, the presence of multiple diagnoses, similar categories were grouped so that six types of disorders were defined: depressive/dysphoric disorders (major depression, minor depression, intermittent depression, labile personality, cyclothymic personality), manic disorders (mania, hypomanic disorder), schizophrenic disorders (schizophrenia, schizoaffective disorder, depressed and manic), anxiety disorders (obsessive compulsive, generalized anxiety, panic, phobic), alcoholism, and personality disorders (antisocial, Briquet's, schizotypal features). Using this system, 13 percent had no disorders, 35 percent had one category of disorder, 31 percent had two, 16 percent had three, and 5 percent had four or five.

DISCUSSION

The most striking finding of this study was that 70.3 percent of our sample of opiate addicts had a current psychiatric disorder and 86.9 percent met diagnostic criteria for at least one psychiatric disorder other than drug abuse at some time in their lives. Moreover, over half (52 percent) had two or more diagnoses in addition to drug abuse. These rates are far higher than those found in a community sample derived from a survey conducted in the New Haven area where the current rates for any psychiatric disorder were 17.8 percent (Weissman, 1978). The specific disorders in which rates were substantially higher in addicts than in normals include major and minor depression, chronic minor mood disorders (intermittent depression, labile personality, cyclothymic personality), alcoholism, antisocial personality, phobic disorder and generalized anxiety disorder. These higher rates were detected despite the average age of this sample being somewhat lower than that in the New Haven survey, giving the addicts a shorter time at risk for disorders (Weissman, 1978). The great majority of psychiatric disorders in our sample are accounted for by chronic or episodic depressive disorders, antisocial personality and alcoholism.

Our finding that over two thirds of our sample have either chronic or episodic depressive disorders extends previous findings using symptom scales and personality measures (Dorus, 1980; Lehman, 1972; Robins, 1974; Rounsaville, 1979; Steer, 1980; Wieland, 1970; Weissman, 1978) which have indicated that depressive symptoms are common in opiate addicts. Our findings are consistent with the clinical theories of Wurmser (1974) and

Khantzian (1977) who suggest that a central problem for the typical addict is regulation of affect and vulnerability to dysphoria. Regarding this hypothesis, it is noteworthy that dysphoric disorders were differentially associated with all other diagnostic categories except schizophrenic disorders.

The finding that a substantial minority of our sample met criteria for antisocial personality is, if anything, surprisingly low given earlier empirical literature and psychodynamic writings suggesting that the typical addict is sociopathic. Our data suggest, instead, that the typical addict is either chronically depressed or vulnerable to episodic depressions. This seeming contrast may reflect genuine changes in the addict population over time, or differences in the kinds of assessments made. In the current study, relatively stringent criteria were used to define antisocial personality, requiring childhood antisocial behavior in addition to adult antisocial behavior that is judged to be independent of the need to obtain drugs. Hence, many addicts in our sample who have performed repeated antisocial acts did not qualify for a diagnosis of antisocial personality, and this may account for the relatively low rate of this diagnosis in the current study. In addition, the prevalence of antisocial personality among addicts may have been exaggerated in previous studies through use of the MMPI psychopathic deviance scale, an empirically derived instrument from which Astin (1959) has identified five factors: (1) self-esteem, (2) hypersensitivity, (3) social maladjustment, (4) emotional deprivation, and (5) impulse control. Many of the items contained in the self-esteem, hypersensitivity, and emotional deprivation groupings are highly suggestive of depression. Moreover, our data show that antisocial personality and depression are not incompatible, even though the typical view of sociopaths would suggest that they are insulated from dysphoria. As we show elsewhere, in our sample, there was a significant association between dysphoric disorders (primarily depression) and personality disorders (primarily antisocial behavior). Stating a commonly held psychoanalytic view, Bursten (1973) has hypothesized that manipulative character traits serve the purpose of defending against powerful underlying feelings of depression, inferiority and emptiness.

The findings that 13.7 percent of the addicts were in current alcoholic episodes and 34.5 percent were alcoholics some time in their lives, extends previous findings (Belenko, 1979) and underscores the need for multimodality treatment aimed at different types of substance abuse. Other disorders which we found in higher rates than might be expected in the general population, including anxiety disorders, hypomania and schizotypal features, were mild and affected a comparatively small minority of our sample. In addition, the validity of these categories may be limited in addicts due to relatively low diagnostic stability (Rounsaville, 1982). Mania and schizophrenic disorders were diagnosed no more frequently than might be expected in a general population. This finding of no excess of schizophrenia or mania in addicts

seems to contradict speculations (Flemmenbaum, 1974; Kleber, 1978)
suggesting that individuals with these disorders may use opiates to contain
psychotic or manic symptomatology. However, since RDC diagnoses are
based on overt symptomatology, we cannot rule out the possibility suggested
by Kleber and Gold (1978) that early and continued use of narcotics and
other CNS depressants may contain symptomatology and result in comparatively attenuated or masked forms of the disorders. If this were the case, our
findings that a comparatively high number of addicts in our sample had
hypomania (6.6 percent) or schizotypal features (8.4 percent) might be seen
as supporting a view of opiates as partial self-treatment for schizophrenia or
mania. More intensive study of addicts with these mild diagnoses would be
needed to follow up this issue.

Treatment Implications

Our finding that the great majority of addicts have secondary psychiatric
disorders underscores the importance of detecting and treating psychological
conditions in opiate addicts. We will focus this discussion on the three major
categories of diagnosis: depressive disorders, antisocial personality, and
alcoholism.

Regarding depression, numerous studies have suggested the value of
psychological and pharmacological treatments for episodic disorders and a
recent study by Akiskal et al (1980) suggests the value of pharmacotherapy
for selected types of chronic, minor mood disorders. In the two well-designed
studies of tricyclic antidepressants as treatment for depression in opiate addicts,
results are mixed with one study showing superiority of tricyclic over placebo
and the other showing no difference (Woody, 1975; Kleber, 1982). Moreover,
a high dropout rate from studies evaluating antidepressant pharmacotherapy in
addicts has also been found in several centers (Edward Khantzian, M.D.,
personal communication) highlighting the problem of using pharmacotherapy
for many addicts who are depressed. With this in mind, studies under way
are testing out the value of individual psychotherapy for opiate addicts.

The finding of a substantial number of addicts with alcoholism suggests
the importance of coordinating drug and alcohol programs, which are usually
administered separately and of incorporating techniques usually reserved to
alcohol treatment in drug treatment programs.

Regarding the substantial minority of our addicts with antisocial
personality, there is no specific treatment for this type of patient. Moreover,
research in personality change in drug treatment has shown that psychopathic
traits do not change even when changes are detected in other characteristics
such as locus of control and depression (DeLeon, 1973; Sutker, 1974;
Rounsaville, 1980). Nevertheless, knowing the diagnosis may help alert the

clinician to the need for definition of rules and limit setting for patients with this disorder.

Diagnosis is only a first step toward effective treatment. Our findings suggest that most addicts have secondary psychiatric disorders. Further work will be needed to develop effective means of treating various diagnostic subgroups. Although the precise treatment implications of a given psychiatric disorder may be unclear, it is clear that adequate diagnosis is necessary in order to call attention to the full range of the addict's problems. Systematic assessment of psychopathology should be incorporated into drug programs.

The system used in the current study, the Schedule for Affective Disorder and Schizophrenia, coupled with the Research Diagnostic Criteria, has much to recommend it as a means of accurately and inexpensively detecting psychiatric disorders. If carefully trained, drug counselors could use the system. As we have shown elsewhere, non-physicians using the SADS were more likely to detect psychiatric disorders than psychiatrists using an open ended interview and the DSM III criteria (Rounsaville, 1980). Moreover, although it does not contain as wide a range of diagnoses as the DSM III, a range of the more important diagnoses is covered.

REFERENCES

Akiskal HS, Rosenthal TL, Haykal RF, Lemmi H, Rosenthal RH and Scott-Strauss A: Characterological depressions: Clinical sleep EEG finding separating "subaffective dysthymias" from "character spectrum disorders." *Arch Gen Psychiat* 37: 777-783, 1980

Astin AW: A factor study of the MMPI Psychopathic Deviate Scale. *J Consult Psychol* 23:550-554, 1959

Barthko JJ and Carpenter WT: On the methods and theory of reliability. *J Nerv Ment Dis* 163:307-317, 1976

Belenko S: Alcohol abuse by heroin addicts: A review of research findings and issues. *Int J Addict* 14:965-975, 1979

Bursten B: Some narcissistic personality types. *Int J Psychoanal* 54:287-300, 1973

Craig RJ: Personality characteristics of heroin addicts: A review of the empirical literature and critique–Part II. *Inter J Addict* 14:607-626, 1979

DeLeon G, Skodal A and Rosenthal MS: Phoenix House: Changes in psychopathological signs of resident drug addicts. *Arch Gen Psychiat* 28:131-135, 1973

Dorus W and Senay EC: Depression, demographic dimensions, and drug abuse. *Am J Psychiatry* 137:699-704, 1980

Endicott J and Spitzer RL: A diagnostic interview: The Schedule for Affective Disorders and Schizophrenia. *Arch Gen Psychiat* 37:837-844, 1978

Flemmenbaum A: Affective disorders and chemical dependence: Lithium for alcohol and drug addiction. *Dis Nerv Syst* 35:281-286, 1974

Hekimian LJ and Gershon S: Characteristics of drug abusers admitted to a psychiatric hospital. *JAMA* 205:75-80, 1968

Khantzian EJ: The ego, the self and opiate addiction: Theoretical and treatment considerations. In: Blaine JD and Julius EA (eds.) *Psychodynamics of Drug Dependence.* National Institute of Drug Abuse Research Monograph 12. U.S. Department of Health, Education and Welfare, Washington, DC, 1977 pp 101–116

Kleber HD and Gold MS: Use of psychotropic drugs in the treatment of methadone maintained narcotic addicts. *Annual of New York Academy of Sciences* 331: 81–98, 1978

Kleber HD, Weissman MM and Rounsaville BJ: Evaluation of psychotherapy in treating heroin dependent individuals. Protocol for NIDA contract. Rockville, MD: 1977

Kleber HD, Weissman MM, Rounsaville BJ and Wilber CH: The treatment of depressed opiate addicts with imipramine. In preparation.

Lehman WX and DeAngelis GG: Adolescents, methadone and psychotherapeutic agents. In: National Association for the Prevention of Addiction to Narcotics. *Proceedings of the Fourth National Conference on Methadone Treatment.* New York: The Association, 1972 pp 55–58

Ling W, Holmes ED, Post GR and Litaker MB: A systematic psychiatric study of the heroin addicts. In: National Association for the Prevention of Addiction to Narcotics. *Proceedings of the Fifth National Conference on Methadone Treatment.* New York: The Association, 1973 pp 429–432

Robins PR: Depression and drug addiction. *Psychoanal Q* 48:375–386, 1974

Rounsaville BJ, Cacciola J, Weissman MM and Kleber HD: Stability of psychiatric diagnoses in opiate addicts. Submitted.

Rounsaville BJ, Rosenberger P, Wilber CH and Weissman MM: Comparison of the SADS/RDC and the DSM-III: Diagnosing drug abusers. *J Nerv Ment Dis* 168: 90–97, 1980

Rounsaville BJ, Weissman MM, Rosenberger PH, Wilber CH and Kleber HD: Detecting depressive disorders in drug abusers: A comparison of screening instruments. *J Affect Dis* 1:255–267, 1979

Sheppard C, Fiorentino D, Collins L and Merlis S: Comparison of emotion profiles as defined by two additional MMPI profile types in male narcotic addicts. *J Clin Psychol* 25:186–188, 1969

Spitzer RL, Endicott J and Robins E: Research Diagnostic Criteria: Rationale and reliability. *Arch Gen Psychiat* 35:773–789, 1978

Steer RA and Kotzker E: Affective changes in male and female methadone patients. *Drug Alcohol Depend* 5:115–122, 1980

Stimmel B: Drug and alcohol treatment. In: Dupont RL, Goldstein A and O'Donnell J (eds) *Handbook on Drug Abuse.* Washington, DC: US Government Printing Office, 1979

Sutker PB, Allain AN and Cohen GH: MMPI indices of personality change following short and long-term hospitalization in heroin addicts. *Psychol Rep* 34:495–500, 1974

Weissman MM and Myers JK: Affective disorders in a United States urban community: The use of Research Diagnostic Criteria in an epidemiological survey. *Arch Gen Psychiat* 35:1304–1314, 1978

Weissman MM, Myers JK and Harding PS: Psychiatric disorders in a United States urban community: 1975–1976. *Am J Psychiat* 135:459–462, 1978

Weissman MM, Slobetz F, Prusoff B, Mesritz M and Howard P: Clinical depression among narcotic addicts maintained on methadone in the community. *Am J Psychiatry* 133:1434–1438, 1976

Wieland WF and Sola S: Depression in opiate addicts measured by objective tests. In: National Association for the Prevention of Addiction to Narcotics. *Proceedings of the Third National Conference on Methadone Treatment.* New York: The Association, 1970

Woody GE, O'Brien CP and Rickels K: Depression and anxiety in heroin addicts: A placebo controlled study of doxepin in combination with methadone. *Am J Psychiat* 132:447–450, 1975

Wurmser L: Psychoanalytic considerations of the etiology of compulsive drug use. *Am Psychoanal Assoc* 22:820–843, 1974

Zimmering P, Toolan J, Safrin R and Wortis SB: Drug addiction in relation to problems of adolescence. Read at the 108th annual meeting of The American Psychiatric Association. Atlantic City, NJ: May 12–16, 1952

Zuckerman M and Sola S: MMPI patterns in drug abusers before and after treatment in therapeutic communities. *J Consult Clin Psychol* 43:286–296, 1975

14

Psychiatric Disorders in Treated Addicts: Discussion

GEORGE E. WOODY

The findings of Drs. Rounsaville, Kleber, and Weissman about psychiatric illnesses in opiate dependent patients are supported by work done in other programs. We have participated in a study funded by the National Institute of Drug Abuse that has done similar diagnostic evaluations on methadone maintained patients, as have Drs. Treece and Khantzian in Boston. Using the SADS-L (the same instrument used by Rounsaville et al), each group found similar results: approximately 25 percent of patients on methadone maintenance have a diagnosis of antisocial personality as defined by the RDC criteria; about 30 percent are suffering a diagnosable depressive illness (either major, minor or intermittent depressive disorder) and about 50 percent have a history of having suffered a depressive disorder at some time in their life. Between 10 and 15 percent have a current anxiety disorder (most commonly generalized anxiety disorder, phobic disorder or obsessive compulsive disorder) and about 15 percent have a current diagnosis of alcoholism. A variety of other diagnoses were found, but these were the most common (1981). The similarity between the findings of Drs. Rounsaville et al and those of the Boston group indicates that these disorders are common and occur with predictable frequency at least among narcotic addicts who are treated in publicly funded programs in these three cities. In addition to these specific problems, a very high proportion of patients had either a current or past history of any kind of psychiatric illness. As mentioned by Dr. Rounsaville, about 85 percent of their patients have a current of past diagnosable psychiatric illness other than substance abuse. These findings support the impression of many clinicians that addicts are a very diverse group when viewed from a psychiatric perspective, and that psychiatric illnesses are seen commonly in substance abuse patients.

These findings also present an opportunity to examine the interface between psychiatric illness and addiction. We have had a special interest in this relationship and have studied it in several ways during the last five years. Some aspects of this relationship which we have observed and which seem important are the following:

First, some of these illnesses can be produced (or perhaps attenuated) by different classes of drugs. McLellan et al recently completed a study of a group of substance abuse patients who had been treated at the inpatient unit of the Coatesville VA Medical Center at least once per year between 1972 and 1978 (1979). Judged by their histories of repeated treatment attempts, these patients had been either treatment failures or were unusually resistant to substance abuse treatment. Every patient had been evaluated psychiatrically by a clinician and was given an MMPI at each admission. These patients were subdivided into three groups, based upon their primary drug of abuse. One group used primarily narcotics, another group used primarily stimulants

Table 1.   Scores and Psychologic Tests in 1972 and 1978

Test	Group 1– 11 Men (Psychostimulants)		Group 2– 14 Men (Psychodepressants)		Group 3– 26 Men (Opiates)	
	1972	1978	1972	1978	1972	1978
SILS						
Mean IQ	101	103	102	94	104	102
Mean cognitive impairment	93	94	93	81	92	91
MMPI*						
Validity	52	54	54	51	56	55
General pathology	64	96†	58	78†	62	66
Hypochondriasis	61	67‡	61	72‡	59	61
Depression	55	58	60	94†	64	66
Hysteria	60	71‡	54	58	54	54
Psychopathy	70	76‡	68	74‡	72	78
Male–female §	64	70	60	58	62	62
Paranoia	63	84†	57	55	59	61
Psychasthenia	56	57	58	62	58	62
Schizophrenia	66	98†	60	63	64	61
Mania	64	87†	63	66	65	59
Social inversion	48	55	55	59	56	58

*MMPI values above 70 indicate severe problem areas.
†$p<0.01$ by paired T-test.
‡$p<0.05$ by paired T-test.
§Inappropriate gender identification.

(amphetamines, cocaine), and a third used mainly sedative type drugs (diazepam, barbiturates, synthetic sedative hypnotics). Each of these groups had similar psychiatric pictures when first seen in 1972—both the MMPI scores and clinical evaluations showed no significant differences at their first admission. But when followed over a six-year period, the stimulant abusers developed a very high proportion of schizophrenic-like symptoms and at the last follow-up point, about 25 percent of these patients had been in long-term psychiatric treatment. The sedative abusers developed a very high proportion of depression. Approximately 30 percent of these had made a suicide attempt and over half were moderately to severely depressed upon examination at their six-year follow-up point. Both the MMPI testing and the psychiatric evaluations were done 10 to 14 days after admission to the unit, so the evaluations did not represent acute drug effects. Interestingly the narcotic dependent patients did not seem to change. When first seen in 1972, they had moderately elevated levels of depression and sociopathic behavior, problems which have traditionally been found in this population. When followed up in subsequent years and in 1978 at the six-year point, this group was approximately the same as upon their first admission.

The most likely explanation for these findings seems to be that the persistent and repeated use of stimulant drugs produced schizophrenic-like

Table 2. Background Variables—Distribution Characteristics

Variable	N	Mean	Standard Deviation
Age	82	31.74	4.60
Education	82	12.02	1.32
Substance Abuse			
Years of regular alcohol intoxication	82	1.52	4.03
Years of regular opiate use	82	8.10	3.95
Years of regular barbiturate use	82	1.01	2.43
Years of regular sedative use	82	1.57	2.86
Years of regular amphetamine use	82	1.24	2.57
Drug treatments	82	3.88	3.07
Drug detoxifications	82	1.95	2.50
Legal			
Serious crimes	82	5.59	7.49
Psychological			
Psychiatric hospitalizations	81	0.65	1.64
Beck	82	14.17	8.44
Shipley C.Q.	78	86.18	15.72
Shipley I.Q.	78	102.08	9.31
Maudsley extroversion	81	26.46	7.21
Maudsley neuroticism	81	26.86	13.22
Symptom checklist	67	67.46	47.91

Table 3. Outcomes of Random Assignment into Cognitive-Behavioral (CB), Supportive-Expressive (SE), or Counselling Alone (DC) Groups

Variable	SE Start	SE 6-Mo	SE 12-Mo	CB Start	CB 6-Mo	CB 12-Mo	DC Start	DC 6-Mo	DC 12-Mo	BGD Start	BGD 6-Mo	BGD 12-Mo
N		11			12			15				
Medical Sev.	1.2	1.5	1.1	2.5	2.5	2.2	2.6	2.7	3.6	+	–	+
Employment Sev.	5.4	3.3	3.2	4.9	4.1	4.5	4.8	4.4	4.8	–	–	–
Days worked	4.2+	13.2*	16.0	3.0+	12.7	9.4	5.1	7.1	9.8	–	+	–
Money earned	216+	560*	805	301	383	345	189	258	247	–	+	+
Drug Sev.	6.4*	2.9	4.3	6.6+	3.6+	3.5	6.6+	3.5	4.5	–	–	–
Days drinking	11.1	6.6	6.0	8.6	5.3+	4.3	9.1	6.3	8.7	–	+	–
Days drunk	3.2*	0.2	1.0	2.8+	0.7+	0.5	3.5	2.3	3.9	–	*	+
Days opiates	14.4*	0.8*	3.7	17.2+	4.5*	1.9	16.4+	3.6*	2.4	–	*	–
Days non opiates	8.1+	2.1	6.8	6.0+	2.0	4.4	6.4	3.8	5.8	–	–	–
Legal Sev.	4.4+	1.8	2.5	5.0+	2.1+	2.1	4.1	2.4	2.8	–	–	–
Crime days	8.6+	1.9	6.1	9.4+	2.1+	4.2	5.1	3.5	5.6	–	*	–
Illegal money	291*	88	236	364+	236*	109	384+	244+	253	–	*	+
Psychological Sev.	3.1	2.1	2.7	3.1	2.6	2.6	3.2	2.9	4.0	–	–	–
Beck	14.1+	8.0	10.1	16.6	9.5	9.9	12.8	11.8	13.7	–	–	+
SCL-90	66.2+	39.6+	29.5	64.2+	34.7+	26.5	58.4	54.4	34.7	–	+	+
Maud-N	28.3	23.8	22.4	29.4+	20.9	24.4	27.6	28.7	29.6	–	+	–
Days in Controlled Environment	5.3	5.4+	1.0	6.2	4.2+	1.7	6.8+	11.5	6.1	–	+	*

+$p < .05$.
*$p < .01$.

disorders in a significant proportion of the patients who were abusing them. Schizophrenic-like illnesses are a well-known acute effect of stimulant use, thus it makes sense that chronic use can produce a persistent schizophrenic-like illness in patients who repeatedly use them. Similarly, persistent use of depressant drugs seemed to produce depression. Again, this is not inconsistent with the pharmacological effects of depressant drugs. Interestingly, there was a lowering of the IQ in the sedative abusers at the 1978 follow-up when compared to the 1972 evaluation. This would indicate that some brain damage had occurred as a result of the sedative drug abuse. Again, this is consistent with reports in the literature showing evidence of neurological impairment in patients who persistently abuse sedatives.

Some of the most striking results of this study were the lack of development of psychiatric disorders in the opiate group. This would indicate that the opiates are relatively non-toxic in terms of their ability to produce major psychiatric disorders. In fact, the possibility exists that opiates may have a modulating or stabilizing effect, and thus may help suppress the emergence of psychiatric disorders (Comfort, 1977). Again, this psychotropic effect of opiates is consistent with the observed pharmacological effects of these drugs, and it has been mentioned as one reason that leads some patients to use narcotics. Table 1 summarizes the findings of this study.

The second point is that a general measure of psychiatric severity taken upon admission to treatment appears to correlate with several measures of outcome. Those patients who had the most severe psychiatric problems upon entering treatment appear to do the worst, and those with the least severe problems do the best (McLellan, 1981).

The third important point is that the amount of current drug use probably correlates with the severity of psychiatric symptoms. The data upon which this statement is based comes from a study that we have been doing in which we are looking at the results obtained by using psychotherapy done by trained professionals when combined with counselling services in a methadone treatment program. This study is one in which patients are randomly assigned to receive either counselling plus cognitive-behavioral (CB),

Table 4. Psychological Status of the Four Groups at the Start of the Study

	High-Sev. Counselling	Low-Sev. Counselling	High-Sev. Therapy	Low-Sev. Therapy
N	10	11	11	10
Beck	18	10	21	9
Maudsley-N	41	24	37	20
Shipley IQ	100	102	96	104
Shipley CQ	80	87	80	94
ASI Psych. Sev.	5.1	2.7	5.6	2.3

or supportive-expressive (SE), psychotherapy, or counselling alone (DC). All
patients entering the study are given a thorough evaluation including the
SADS-L with RDC and DSM-III diagnoses; social, legal, medical, family and
vocational evaluations; and measures of current psychiatric symptoms such as
the SCL-90, the Beck, and the SADS-C. Our preliminary results indicate that
the patients who were randomly assigned to receive psychotherapy in addition
to counselling are doing better as measured by urine test results, methadone
dosage, prescribed medications, and other measures of outcome. These
results are summarized in Tables 2 and 3 and Figures 1, 2, and 3.

When we separate patients who received counselling or counselling plus
psychotherapy into those who have high and low levels of psychiatric severity,
we find the following results, summarized in Tables 4 and 5 and Figures 4, 5,
and 6.

As seen in the tables and figures, patients who were judged by the
criteria listed in Table 4 to have high or low levels of psychiatric symptoms
used correspondingly higher or lower amounts of medication as judged doses
of methadone, urine test results and prescriptions for ancillary medicines.
Thus, we see a relationship between psychiatric severity and both prescribed
and unprescribed drug use. Interestingly, we find that both the psychotherapy
and the counselling groups who had low levels of psychiatric severity
benefitted about equally from the treatment programs. However, patients
with high levels of psychiatric severity appeared to receive minimal benefit

Table 5. Pre- to Post-Therapy Improvement

	High-Sev. Counselling		Low-Sev. Counselling		High-Sev. Therapy		Low-Sev. Therapy	
N	10		11		11		10	
Medical Sev.	3.1	2.4	1.7	3.2	2.5	3.5	1.8	0.7
Days med. probs.	4	2	2	4	3	3	1	1
Employment Sev.	4.5	4.6	5.1+	3.2	3.8	3.0	3.9+	2.7
Days worked	9	11	10	13	7	10	9	13
Money earned	272	306	242+	380	309+	482	318*	523
Abuse Sev.	5.7+	3.8	3.8*	1.4	4.9+	3.0	4.0*	1.4
Days drunk	4	2	2	1	3	2	2	0
Days opiate	6	3	10*	2	5	2	8+	3
Days nonopiate	10	8	4	2	7+	3	3	1
Money for drugs	430*	190	164*	47	344*	65	188*	8
Legal Sev.	3.1	3.0	4.5+	3.1	2.8+	0.7	2.0+	0.8
Days crime	6	3	10+	4	5+	0.8	1	0.4
Illegal income	216	181	506+	300	186*	43	166*	10
Psychological Sev.	5.1	4.8	2.7	1.8	5.6+	3.0	2.5+	1.0
Days psych. probs.	17	13	8	3	15+	8	4+	1

*p<.01.
+p<.05.

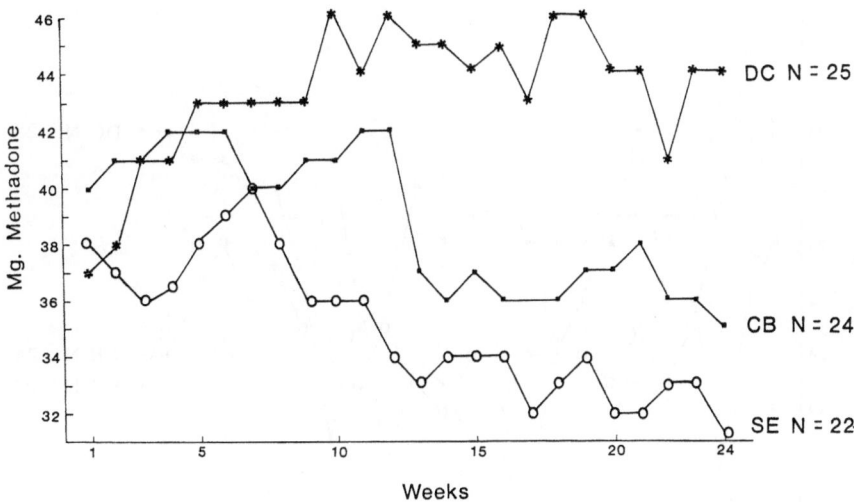

Fig. 1. Methadone dose.

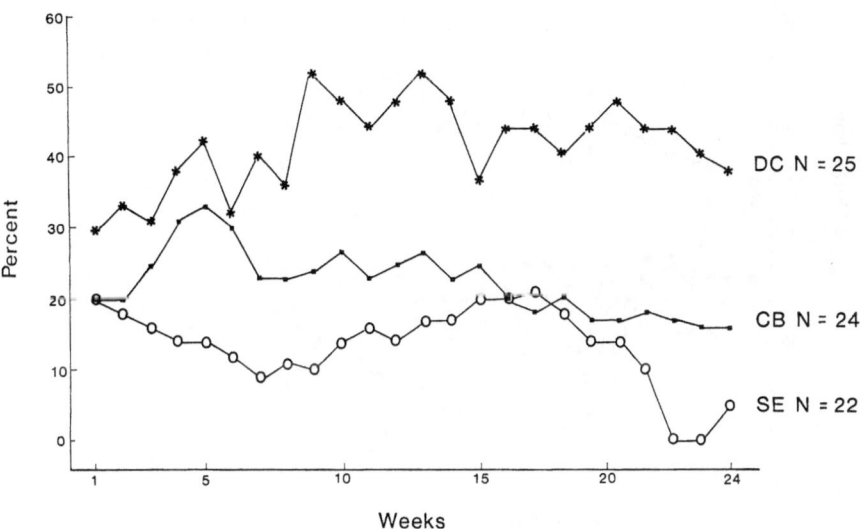

Fig. 2. Patients receiving ancillary medications.

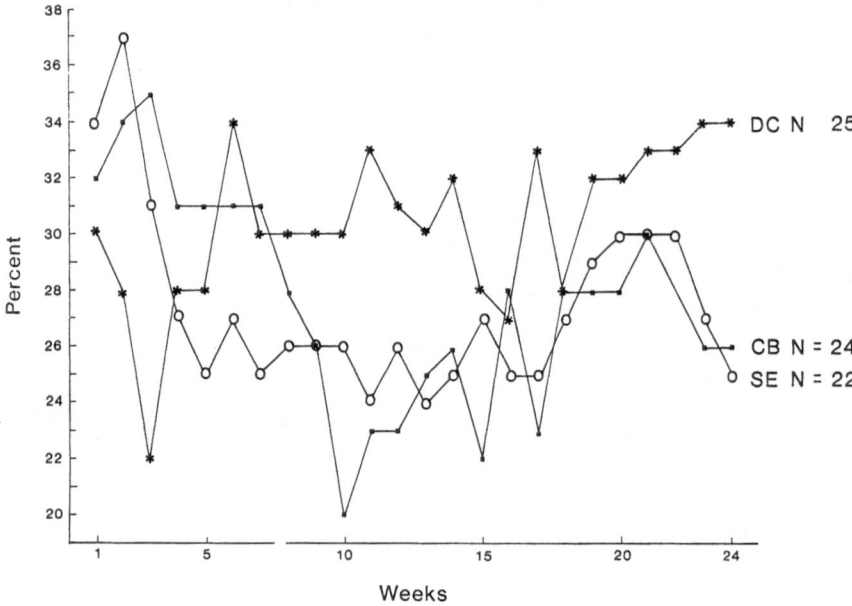

Fig. 3. Positive urines.

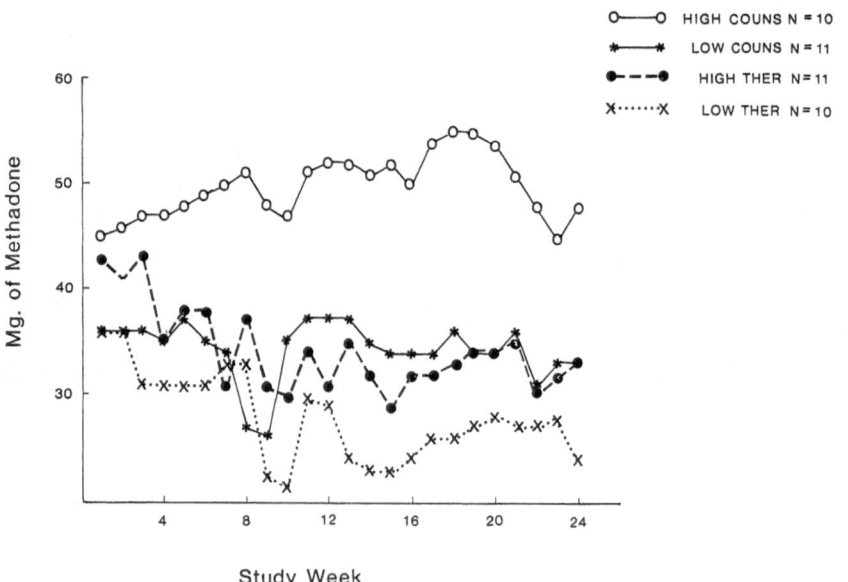

Fig. 4. Mean methadone dosage by group.

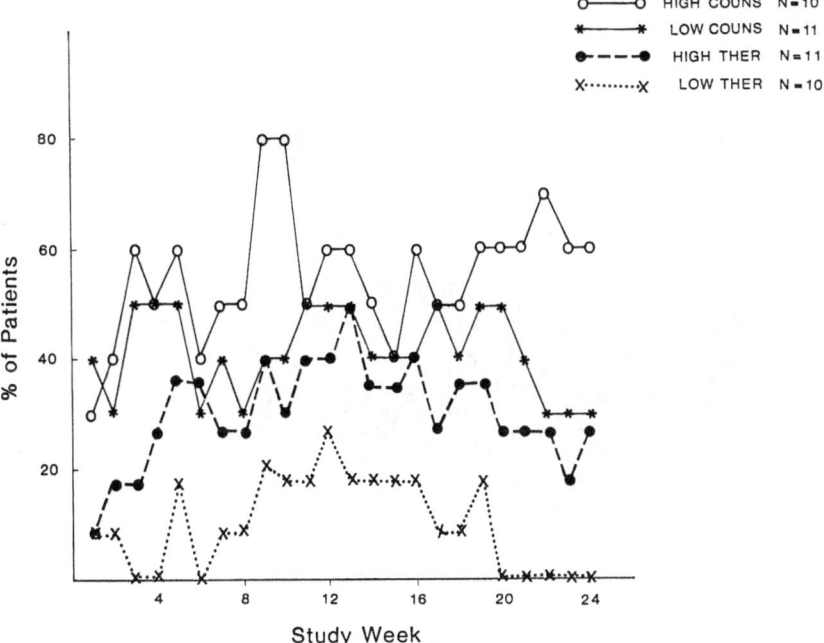

Fig. 5. Patients receiving ancillary medication by group.

from counselling alone whereas they seemed to receive significant benefits from the combination of counselling and psychotherapy. This finding can be of practical interest. Patients with high levels of psychiatric severity may benefit by the use of more highly trained personnel when treated in a methadone program, and they may not improve much unless they receive this extra help. Those with relatively low levels of psychiatric symptoms seem to do well with the routine clinical services and it is probably not necessary to add special treatments for these patients.

Implications: These findings have several implications. One is that illicit drugs use may represent attempts to self-medicate psychiatric symptoms for some patients. For these particular patients, psychiatric problems can contribute to the severity and perhaps to the continuation of the addiction. Insofar as addicts are psychiatrically impaired, which many seem to be, psychiatric illnesses may be important contributors to addiction. The frequency of drug use itself does not seem to be an important determinant of outcome. A second implication is that the choice of drug may play a significant role in determining whether the person remains stable (or perhaps becomes more integrated), or

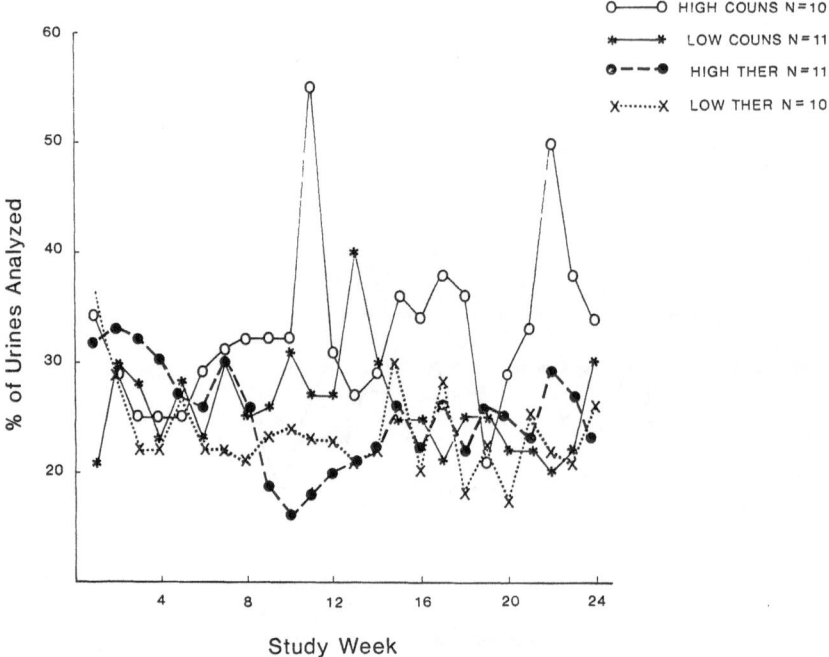

Fig. 6. Positive urines by group.

becomes more disorganized. Here I am referring to the study by McLellan et al in which patients who used sedatives and stimulants developed psychiatric illnesses whereas those who used opiates did not. The last implication is that diagnosis and effective treatment of psychiatric problems, along with other services (such as legal counselling, vocational interventions and appropriate pharmacological support) may improve outcome, especially in patients with high degrees of psychiatric severity.

REFERENCES

Comfort A: Morphine as an antipsychotic: Relevance of a 19th-century therapeutic fashion. *Lancet* 2:448–449, 1977
McLellan AT, Luborsky L, Woody GE, O'Brien CP and Kron R: Are the "addiction-related" problems of substance abusers really related? *The Journal of Nervous and Mental Disease* 169:232–239, 1981

McLellan AT, Woody GE and O'Brien CP: Development of psychiatric illness in drug
    abusers. *N Eng J Med* 301:1310–1314, 1979
Nace EP, O'Brien CP, Mintz J, Ream N and Meyers AL: Adjustment among Vietnam
    veterans drug users: Two years post service. In: Figley CP, PhD (ed) *Stress
    Disorders Among Vietnam Veterans.* Brunner/Mazel: New York, 1978 pp 71–128
Reported at project review meeting held by NIDA. Parklawn Building, Rockville, Md.
    January 24, 1981

15

Naltrexone: Current Clinical Investigations

HAROLD M. GINZBURG
ROBERT A. MARKOWITZ

The National Institute on Drug Abuse (NIDA) has the lead governmental role in developing New Chemical Entities (NCEs) into chemotherapeutic agents for the treatment of drug abuse. The Alcohol, Drug Abuse, and Mental Health Administration (ADAMHA) and its sister agency the National Institutes of Health (NIH) jointly share the difficult task of developing agents of little commercial value that are termed orphan drugs. NIDA has identified several substances as being both safe and efficacious in the treatment of opioid abuse. We focus on the process involved in transforming an NCE, EN-1639A (naltrexone), into a chemotherapeutic agent with a New Drug Application (NDA) approved by the Food and Drug Administration (FDA). In addition, specific data that were collected during delays in this process are presented, and the use of this data base to facilitate the NDA process is discussed.

In order to place these clinical data on naltrexone in a proper perspective, it is necessary to present (1) an overview of the FDA process, (2) an historical perspective of narcotic antagonists, and (3) a discussion of factors contributing to the delay of the scheduled Phase III studies, and the resultant implication.

THE FOOD AND DRUG ADMINISTRATION

The FDA is mandated to review preclinical and clinical material developed on new chemical entities to determine whether or not they will be safe and efficacious agents in the treatment of recognized medical conditions.

157

A comprehensive set of preclinical and clinical guidelines has been developed and implemented as a result of experiences with other chemotherapeutic agents, including the ill-fated thalidomide experience.

There are four types of preclinical studies which must be conducted. One requirement is that these investigations must include data derived from at least two different animal species. Furthermore, it is required that control and experimental groups of sufficient size be used to permit statistical evaluation of the results. Four categories of preclinical investigations include:

1. Short term toxicity studies to determine LD-50s, effects on food and water intake, gross behavior, mortality, and other relevant information.
2. Two-year carcinogenicity studies with observations of gross behavior, and gross and microscopic tissue examinations.
3. Two-year chronic toxicity studies with metabolic, enzymatic, growth, and development examinations.
4. Reproduction and teratology studies:
   (a) Study of fertility and general reproductive performance—Emphasis is on the effects of a given drug on gonadal function, estrous cycles, mating behavior, conception rates, and the early stages of gestation.
   (b) Teratological study—Emphasis is on determining whether a drug has a potential for embryotoxicity and/or teratogenicity; drug administration is restricted to the period of organogenesis.
   (c) Perinatal and postnatal study—Emphasis is on the effects of a drug administered during the last trimester of pregnancy and the period of lactation.

There are three clinical phases in the development of an NDA. These are:

Phase I: Pharmacology studies are used to determine toxicity, metabolism, absorption, and elimination, and other pharmacological actions; preferred route of administration, and safe dosage range are also studied. These studies involve a small number of persons and are conducted under carefully controlled circumstances by persons trained in clinical pharmacology. Approximately 20 to 80 healthy, male volunteer subjects participate in this phase which lasts approximately 9–12 months.

Phase II: Initial clinical trials are conducted on a limited number of patients to evaluate the agent and its effectiveness in the prevention or treatment of a specific disease. Additional pharmacological studies performed concurrently on animals may be necessary to further evaluate safety. The closely monitored human clinical trials designed to demonstrate efficacy and relative safety generally involve between

100 and 200 patients. This phase takes approximately two years to complete.

Phase III: Proposals for this phase involving extensive clinical trials are in order if the information obtained in the first two phases demonstrates reasonable assurance of safety and effectiveness, or suggests that the drug may have a potential value outweighing possible hazards. The Phase III studies are intended to assess the drug's safety, effectiveness, and most desirable dosage in treating a specific disease in a large group of subjects. These studies may vary considerably with respect to extent but are in any case carefully monitored. They usually do not exceed three years in total length.

The FDA is regularly provided with updated reports on the progress of each phase. If the continuation of the studies appears to present an unwarranted hazard to the patients/subjects, the sponsor may be requested to modify or discontinue clinical testing until further preclinical work has been done (Tocus, 1976).

HISTORICAL PERSPECTIVE ON NARCOTIC ANTAGONISTS

Wikler's work with narcotic antagonists during the 1960s (Wikler, 1965) was further pursued by Martin et al (1967) at NIDA's Addiction Research Center, Lexington, Kentucky. It was demonstrated that narcotic antagonists could be effectively used to block the euphoria and dependence producing properties of opioids. Most significantly, these chemotherapeutic agents did not have pronounced behavioral effects as was the case with methadone, did not produce either physical or psychological dependence, and thus could be characterized as having no abuse liability.

The current theories of blockade of opioids by the narcotic antagonists are based on the physical mechanism of competitive inhibition. Antagonists occupy the same receptor sites as agonists but have little or no intrinsic activity at those sites. The optimal characteristics of narcotic antagonists should include the following properties (Julius, 1976):

1. Ability to antagonize the euphoria produced by the opioids;
2. Absent or low agonist effects, especially unpleasant effects;
3. Do not cause physical dependence;
4. Tolerance to the antagonistic actions does not develop;
5. Absence of serious side effects and toxicity with acute and chronic use;
6. Easily administered, preferably by the oral route;
7. Duration of action sufficient to require daily or less frequent administration;

8. Absent (or low) abuse potential;
9. Reversible effects, in case of medical emergency;
10. High potency to allow administration of small amounts in a biodegradable vehicle;
11. Easily available and relatively inexpensive;
12. High level of patient acceptance.

In the search for a chemical entity possessing these characteristics, narcotic antagonists, including naloxone (Blumberg et al, 1961), nalorphine (Eckenhoff et al, 1952), cyclazocine (Jaffe, 1967), and naltrexone (Julius and Renault, 1976) have been evaluated for potential clinical use. Naloxone was the first narcotic antagonist discovered that was virtually devoid of all agonistic activity (Foldes et al, 1969). It is reported to be a competitive antagonist at the mu, kappa, and sigma receptors. Foldes et al (1963) demonstrated naloxone to be an efficacious chemotherapeutic agent in man. Jasinski et al (1967) determined that when naloxone was administered chronically, and in large dosages, it did not produce physical dependence, further demonstrating its lack of agonist effects. Naloxone has limited clinical use as a less than chronic narcotic antagonist because of its relatively short half-life and the necessity for parenteral administration (Zaks et al, 1971). Naloxone, however, has become a standard pharmacologic agent for use to reverse the respiratory depression frequently associated with opioid overdose. Virtually all agonist effects induced by any opioid can be reversed by naloxone. Its ability to induce an immediate withdrawal syndrome makes naloxone particularly useful in the diagnosis of opioid dependence (Judson et al, 1980).

Cyclazocine (Resnick et al, 1970) was reported to be a promising longer acting antagonist. The duration of action of a 4 mg dose was reported to be as long as 24 hours. However, dysphoria and psychotomimetic effects were unacceptable concommitant reactions (Resnick et al, 1971). Although the development of tolerance to these side effects was clinically documented, cyclazocine was not well received by the volunteer addicts and subsequent clinical populations who were offered this chemotherapeutic agent.

Blumberg and Dayton (1973) reported that EN-1639A seemed to be a potent antagonist that did not produce either the dysphoria or other unpleasant side effects of cyclazocine. The reported duration of narcotic blockade following oral administration of 50 mg was 24 hours. Martin (Martin and Jasinski, 1973; Martin et al, 1973) and Resnick et al (1974a,b,c) suggested that naltrexone (EN-1639A), fulfilled the criteria of an optimal narcotic antagonist. In 1973, the NIDA initiated and funded a series of preclinical and clinical research studies to further elucidate the safety and efficacy of naltrexone. The preclinical studies were designed to meet the FDA requirements for the eventual approval of an NDA permitting clinical researchers to dispense naltrexone according to a reviewed and approved protocol. A number of studies were simultaneously undertaken, involving clinical researchers in more than a dozen clinics; however, not all researchers used the same protocol. Five clinics did participate in a double blind placebo controlled study of naltrexone conducted by the National Academy of Sciences (Committee on the Clinical Evaluation of Narcotic Antagonists, unpublished observations). Controlled and uncontrolled clinical trials were undertaken by Brahen et al (1976), Lewis (1975), O'Brien et al (1975), and others (Schecter, 1975; Taintor et al, 1975). Almost all investigators used a total weekly dose of 350 mg, liquid, on a three times weekly basis (100 mg Mondays, 100 mg Wednesdays, 150 mg Fridays) except Brahen who administers naltrexone twice weekly (150 mg Mondays, 200 mg Thursdays).

Some researchers terminated their use of naltrexone after the funding ceased. However, a number of researchers, including Brahen, Czertko, O'Brien, Resnick, and others continued to administer naltrexone to clients following the protocols developed for the Phase II study despite the lack of supplemental Federal research funds. Brahen (Nassau County Department of Drug and Alcohol Addiction Program) has, at this point, administered naltrexone to over 550 clients in a program with a voluntary Antagonist Treatment Unit and a prison Work-Release Unit.

THE DELAY, ITS CAUSES, AND ITS IMPLICATIONS

During the initial review of the early progress reports from the naltrexone carcinogenicity studies, some of the preliminary data suggested that naltrexone might have the potential of being carcinogenic. This occurred immediately prior to the commencement of the Phase III clinical studies. At this point, NIDA ordered that Phase III not commence until the animal studies were completed and the animal tissues reviewed by independent pathologists. Existing clients were permitted to continue on naltrexone, and new clients were permitted to be inducted and maintained on naltrexone. In both cases, clients were given an informed consent form which clearly stated that naltrexone might have the potential of being a carcinogen, but stated that the client had to consider the clinical benefits from the substance, and weigh them against the risks. It should be noted that the Drug Abuse Reporting Program (DARP) had established the death rate of clients continuing to use heroin or other opioids at approximately 1.5 percent per year (Watterson et al, 1974). This death rate, and it is assumed, comparably high morbidity rate, is at least ten times greater than the anticipated age specific rates.

The large scale clinical trials were to have been initiated two years ago. However, understandably, ENDO Laboratories, Inc., the pharmaceutical firm developing naltrexone, and the Government, were unwilling to continue extensive human testing until resolution of the carcinogenicity issue occurred. The final carcinogenicity reports were reviewed by outside independent consultants in September 1980 (Braude, 1980). Several independent review groups studied the findings and issued a statement which in essence indicated that, based on the Mason Research Institute (MRI) data, there was no evidence to conclude that naltrexone was a carcinogenic agent in the species of animals tested.

ENDO and the government were now in the position to initiate the Phase III studies. The decision on how to proceed was not as simple as it might have appeared. The contract to conduct the Phase III studies was in place, and the contractor was ready and eager to commence data collection. At this point, it was recognized that a number of researchers and clinicians had continued to collect data on clients maintained on naltrexone, and that the format of the data was the same as had been used in the earlier Phase II clinical studies and would be used in Phase III studies. Therefore, an initial exploration of these data was made to determine whether they were sufficient to provide the basis for an approvable NDA, thus obviating the necessity for carrying out the complete Phase III studies as initially conceived. The data that are presented below are based on the client records of the Nassau County Outpatient Drug Abuse Treatment Programs (Table 1). Over 550 clients were inducted on naltrexone without serious adverse sequelae. Almost all

Table 1. Demographic Data on Clients in the Voluntary Naltrexone Program and the Prison Work Release Program

	Voluntary Program (n=100)	Work Release Program (n=172)	All Clients* (n=287)
Demographic Variable			
Sex			
Male	87%	96.5%	93.4%
Female	13	3.5	6.6
Race/ethnic			
White	79%	35.5%	52.3%
Black	20	61	45.3
Hispanic	1	3.5	2.4
Mean age	29 years	28 years	28 years
Age range	21–48	19–53	19–53
Criminal justice related referral	30%	100%	
Mean number of urines screened per client	27 urines	59 urines	54 urines
Range of urines screened per client	6–213	5–230	5–441
Adverse reactions			
Life-threatening	0	0	0
Non-life-threatening (rash or GI complaint)	1	2	4

*Includes 15 clients that had received treatment in both units.

of the adverse drug reactions reported are related to gastrointestinal upset. It appears that these reactions are the result of a precipitated withdrawal in clients who have not been opiate-free for an adequate length of time. A tablet preparation will be available by late summer 1981; thus, the other subjective complaint, the bitter taste of the liquid preparation, hopefully will be obviated. The only other single adverse drug reaction was the development of a non-life-threatening rash. There was equivocal evidence that the client in question had been concurrently taking unknown substances in addition to the naltrexone.

THE DATA

This data base represents clients that remained in treatment more than six consecutive weeks in either the voluntary Naltrexone Treatment Unit of the Nassau County Drug Abuse Treatment Program or the Work Release Treatment Unit of the Nassau County Jail. Six weeks was arbitrarily selected as the minimum time necessary for a patient to be considered to be engaged in treatment. During the period 1976 to April 1981, approximately 550 clients were inducted on naltrexone in both of these treatment units.

At least 287 clients have been identified as being on naltrexone for a minimum of one six week period, 16 percent had multiple treatment episodes (4.5 percent of all clients or 30 percent of those having a second treatment episode returned for a third). Approximately 200 of the clients in treatment for the minimum six week period have evidence in their records of at least two complete physical examinations and laboratory studies (at admission, and at termination from treatment), meeting the FDA reporting criteria to be considered a "case" in an NDA submission.

One hundred seventy two clients in this sample were from the work release program, 100 from the voluntary outpatient treatment program; an additional 14 clients were initially in the work release program and when they completed that program voluntarily transferred to the outpatient program; one client commenced naltrexone as a voluntary outpatient and continued it as a client of the work release program.

The client population was predominately male (93.4 percent), the mean age was 28 years. In the voluntary program, 79 percent of the clients were white, 20 percent Black and 1 percent Hispanic. In the work release program, 35.5 percent were White, 61 percent Black and 3.5 percent Hispanic.

Thirty-five percent of the voluntary naltrexone treatment unit clients and 37 percent of work release clients did not have a history of prior drug abuse treatment. In almost all cases heroin or another opioid was considered the primary drug of abuse at admission to treatment. Unlike clients entering drug free treatment programs for *nonopioid* related problems, these clients do not deny their drug related problems. What is worthy of note, in the work release program, is that 74 percent of these clients stated that they did not have a drug related problem in the month prior to entrance into the treatment program; all the clients were incarcerated during this period of time. Seventeen percent of the voluntary clients also stated that in the month before treatment their drug use was not a problem; a large proportion of these clients were also either incarcerated or under strict legal supervision during this period. It is, therefore, important to qualify answers which are related to access to drugs, and access to the community.

The results of the urine screening program were most provocative. Sixteen percent of the voluntary clients never had a positive urine for opioids, quinine, barbiturates, cocaine, or amphetamines, and half of all urines that were drug positive were so for only one substance. This does not appear to be a population of multiple substance abusers. Alcohol and marijuana are not considered in this discussion as these substances are relatively ubiquitous in similar age-specific populations not in treatment programs for opiate use.

The results of the urine testing program in the work release program were impressive. Slightly more than 40 percent (42.4 percent) never had a drug positive urine. More than half of the positive urines were for quinine alone. Morphine accounted for less than 10 percent of the positive urines. Whether the incidence of urines positive for quinine reflects heavy gin and tonic consumption, or the use of illicit heroin of poor quality heavily adulterated with quinine, is speculative.

Induction procedures are designed to stabilize clients on a maintenance dose of a chemotherapeutic agent while minimizing the possibility of adverse reactions. These procedures varied markedly between the work release and voluntary outpatient program. Immediate induction to 150 mg of naltrexone was the procedure of choice for the work release program (61 percent), with one week of 50 mg daily dose induction being used half as frequently (32 percent). Both clinics used a twice rather than a three times weekly standard regimen, with 150 mg being administered on Mondays and 200 mg being administered on Thursdays. In the voluntary program, 86 percent were inducted by the one day graduated procedure. Ten mg were given, and if no evidence of withdrawal was seen, additional amounts were given over several hours until a total of 150 mg was administered. Naloxone challenges infrequently were administered. The mean duration of treatment in the work release program was 11 weeks, and in the voluntary program 12 weeks. Ninety-seven percent of the work release clients did not have any lapses of naltrexone intake during their treatment experience; 52 percent of the voluntary clients did (of these 2/3, or 35 percent of the total number of voluntary clients, had only a single lapse). A lapse is defined as missing two consecutive doses of naltrexone, or one week of treatment. A client was considered to have dropped out of treatment after he or she missed eight successive doses of naltrexone, four weeks of treatment. Seven work release clients and 28 voluntary clients had two separate treatment experiences with naltrexone, and eleven voluntary clients (eleven of the 28) had three separate treatment experiences. It is noteworthy that in the voluntary program 15 percent of the clients remained in treatment more than 28 weeks, and that some who have terminated naltrexone continue to be "drug free" and attend the clinic for counseling.

It appears that both the work release clients and the clients in the voluntary program are appropriate candidates for naltrexone treatment. They appear to have had significant involvement with the criminal justice system and most of the clients have had prior treatment experiences. They appear to tolerate the naltrexone with a minimum of adverse side effects. Only four minor adverse reactions were reported in more than 50 patient-years experience provided by almost three hundred clients.

This single data base, fortuitously collected during administrative delays in the development of the NDA for naltrexone could be used as the basis for a limited NDA. These data and the data from other researchers should be sufficient to demonstrate to the FDA that naltrexone is a safe and efficacious drug for at least six weeks of treatment in males with a history of heroin or opioid abuse. Additional research, in the standard Phase III format, will be necessary to provide sufficient short-term data on women and long-term data on both men and women before anticipated unrestricted approval of the NDA by FDA will occur. These necessary studies will commence this year.

It is anticipated that when the FDA grants the limited NDA for naltrexone it will provide the clinician with the discretion of continuing clients on naltrexone for additional six week cycles. If this is not the case, then clinicians will need INDs to provide continuous naltrexone treatment for greater than the approved six week time period.

SUMMARY

This paper has attempted to outline the preclinical and clinical studies necessary to obtain approval of an NDA from the FDA. The particular substance discussed in this paper, EN-1639A, or naltrexone, has been determined to be both efficacious and safe as a chemotherapeutic agent in the treatment of clients with a history of heroin or opioid use and wishing to control their drug seeking behavior. However, because of a number of issues unrelated to the clinical studies, the NDA has been delayed for several years. Clinicians, believing in this drug, have continued to treat clients with it, under their own INDs. The data from one clinic were presented in this paper to indicate the magnitude of available data which may become part of an NDA. These data appear to be sufficient to justify an NDA for limited use (up to six weeks) in males until such time as additional data can be compiled on long term administration in both men and women.

REFERENCES

Blumberg H and Dayton HB: Naloxone, naltrexone, and related noroxymorphones. In: Braude MC, Harris LS, May EL, Smith JP and Villarreal JE (eds) *Narcotic Antagonists.* New York, Raven Press, pp 33–44, 1973

Blumberg H, Dayton HB, George M and Rappaport DN: N-allylnoroxymorphone: A potent narcotic antagonist. *Fed Proc* 20:311, 1961

Brahen LS, Capone T, Weichert V, Babinski A and Desiderio D: A comparison of controlled clinical and laboratory studies of the narcotic antagonists cyclazocine and naltrexone. Presented at the Third National Drug Abuse Conference, New York, March 1976

Braude MC (moderator): *Final Report: Technical Review on Carcinogenicity Studies of Naltrexone.* Rockville, Maryland, The National Institute on Drug Abuse, 1980

Eckenhoff JE, Elder JD and King BD: N-Allyl-normorphine in the treatment of morphine or demerol narcosis. *Am J Med Sci* 223:191–197, 1952

Foldes FF, Duncalf D and Kuwabara S: The respiratory, circulatory, and narcotic antagonistic effects of nalorphine, levallorphan, and naloxone in anaesthetized subjects. *Can Anaesth Soc J* 16:151–161, 1969

Foldes FF, Lunn JN, Moore J and Brown IM: N-allylnoroxymorphone: A new potent narcotic antagonist. *Am J Med Sci* 245:23–30, 1963

Jaffe J: Cyclazocine in the treatment of narcotic addiction. In: Masserman JH (ed) *Current Psychiatric Therapies,* Vol. VII. New York, Grune and Stratton, pp 147–156, 1967

Jasinski DR, Martin WR and Haertzen CA: The human pharmacology and abuse potential of N-allylnoroxymorphone (naloxone). *J Pharmacol Exp Ther* 157: 420–426, 1967

Judson BA, Himmelberger DU and Goldstein A: The naloxone test for opiate dependence. *Clin Pharmacol Ther* 27:492–501, 1980

Julius D: NIDA'S Naltrexone Research Program. In: Julius D and Renault P (eds) *Narcotic Antagonist: Naltrexone.* Washington, DC, National Institute on Drug Abuse Research Monograph 9. DHHS Pub. No. (ADM) 77-387, pp 5–11, 1976

Julius D and Renault P (eds): *Narcotic Antagonists: Naltrexone.* Washington, DC, National Institute on Drug Abuse Research Monograph 9, DHHS Pub. No. (ADM) 77-387, 1976

Lewis DC: The clinical usefulness of narcotic antagonists: Preliminary findings of the use of naltrexone. *Am J Drug Alcohol Abuse* 2:403–415, 1975

Martin WR: Opioid antagonists. *Pharm Rev* 19:463–522, 1967

Martin WR and Jasinski DR: Characterization of EN-1639A. *Clin Pharmacol Ther* 14:142, 1973

Martin WR, Jasinski DR and Mansky PA: Naltrexone, an antagonist for the treatment of heroin dependence effects in man. *Arch Gen Psychiatry* 28:784–791, 1973

O'Brien CP, Greenstein RA, Mintz J and Woody GE: Clinical experience with naltrexone. *Am J Drug Alcohol Abuse* 2:365–377, 1975

Pilot Studies in the Clinical Evaluation of Narcotic Antagonists. Prepared by The Committee on the Clinical Evaluation of Narcotic Antagonists. Division of

Medical Sciences, Assembly of Life Sciences, National Research Council. Washington, DC, 1977 (unpublished)

Resnick R, Fink M and Freedman A: A cyclazocine typology in opiate dependence. *Am J Psychiatry* 126:90–94, March 1970

Resnick R, Fink M and Freedman A: Cyclazocine treatment of opiate dependence: A progress report. *Compr Psychiatry* 12:491–502, 1971

Resnick R, Volavka J and Freedman AM: Short-term effects of naltrexone: A progress report. In: Proceedings of the Committee on Problems of Drug Dependence of the National Academy of Sciences, pp 250–263, 1974

Resnick R, Volavka J, Freedman AM and Thomas M: Studies of EN-1639A (naltrexone): A new narcotic antagonist. *Am J Psychiatry* 131:646–650, 1974

Resnick R, Volavka J, Gaztanaga P and Freedman AM: *Clinical Pharmacology of Naltrexone.* Presented to 9th Congress of the Collegium Internationale Neuropsychopharmacologicum, Paris, July 1974

Schecter A: Clinical use of naltrexone (EN-1639A) Part II: Experience with the first 50 patients in a New York City treatment clinic. *Am J Drug Alcohol Abuse* 2:433–442, 1975

Taintor Z, Landsberg R, Wicks N, Plumb M, D'Amanda C and Greenwood J: Experiences with naltrexone in Buffalo. *Am J Drug Alcohol Abuse* 2:391–401, 1975

Tocus EC: Requirements for drug development. In: Julius D and Renault P (eds) *Narcotic Antagonists: Naltrexone.* Washington, DC, National Institute on Drug Abuse Research Monograph 9. DHHS Publ No. (ADM) 77-387, pp 12–15, 1976

Watterson O, Sells SB and Simpson DD: Death rates and causes of death among opiate addicts in the DARP during 1971–1972. In: Sells SD (ed) *The Effectiveness of Drug Abuse Treatment,* Vol. II. Cambridge, Massachusetts, Ballinger Publishing Company, pp 361–392, 1974

Wikler A: Conditioning factors in opiate addiction and release. In: Wilner DI and Kossebaum GG (eds) *Narcotics.* New York, McGraw Hill, pp 85–100, 1965

Zaks A, Jones T, Fink M and Freedman AM: Naloxone treatment of opiate dependence. *J Am Med Assoc* 215:2108–2110, 1971

16

Clinical Pharmacology and Therapeutic Use of the Narcotic Antagonist: Naltrexone

KARL VEREBEY

INTRODUCTION

Due to the chemical complexity of the human organism it is difficult to imagine that any one chemical agent would produce a single pharmacological effect. The "magic bullet" theory, envisioned by Paul Erlich around the turn of the century, postulated that after drug administration the drug is absorbed, transported by the blood to its site of action, performs the desired pharmacological action without effecting other cells or organs and then excreted. It was soon discovered that such selective chemicals were nonexistent. After searching for decades, scientists had to be satisfied by finding chemicals with the minimal number and least severe side effects. Interestingly, naltrexone seems to be close to the description of the "magic bullet."

Addiction to narcotics occurs after the chronic interaction of the opiate receptors in the brain with the exogenous opioids such as heroin, morphine, or methadone. What happens if the opiates cannot interact with the receptors because they are already occupied by another ligand which has no opioid activity? The answer is: nothing, absolutely nothing, and this is the most desired pharmacological effect of naltrexone. In most ex-addicts naltrexone has no readily observable effects. A way to confirm the presence of naltrexone is by the injection of heroin. This procedure is called a "heroin challenge." If a sufficient amount of naltrexone is present in the individual, all the heroin related effects are blocked. By having a greater affinity for the opiate receptor than heroin, naltrexone is able to interfere with the heroin-opiate receptor interaction and consequently prevent the development or continuation of narcotic addiction. If this is true, we have a perfect drug which could end heroin addiction once and for all. If naltrexone is such a perfect drug, why isn't there more enthusiasm about its development for general use? In this overview of the pharmacodynamics and medical application of naltrexone I will also examine the possible reasons for the relatively low profile of naltrexone.

HISTORY

Martin was the first to suggest using antagonists as a protective measure for ex-opiate addicts to remain abstinent (Martin, 1966). Various compounds were tested for this purpose. Naloxone, the N-allyl congener of naltrexone, is a pure narcotic antagonist with a short time/action. When tested as an opiate blocker, gram quantities were needed to provide 24 hr protection against heroin effects. Not only were the large doses of naloxone uncomfortable for the patients but the large amount needed for continued therapy was very expensive. Another compound, a partial agonist-antagonist, cyclazocine was also tested for the same purpose. This drug at very low doses had a desirable, long duration of narcotic blockade. But in many subjects it caused psychotomimetic reactions especially during induction, which was unacceptable for most subjects (Verebey, 1975).

The synthesis of naltrexone was one of those rare projects in which a logical line of thought was followed resulting exactly in the desired product. Blumberg et al (1965) thought of the possible transplantation of the cyclazocine N-substitution, the cyclopropyl-methyl group, onto the nitrogen of naloxone replacing the allyl group (Fig. 1). The resulting molecule, named

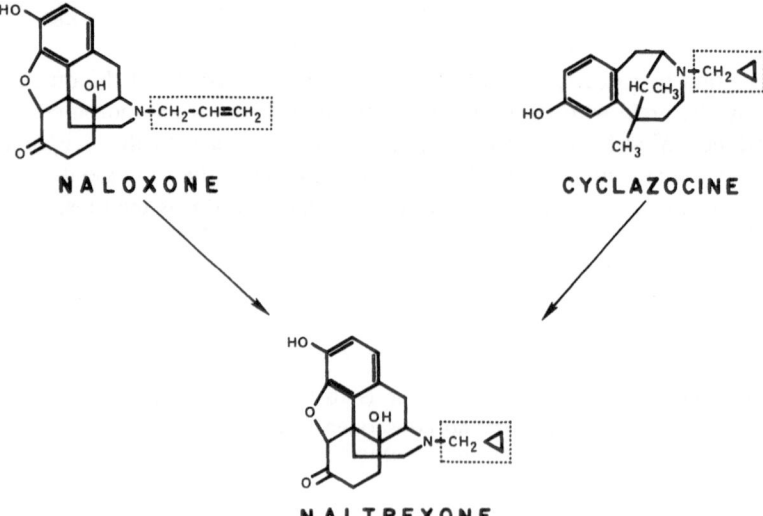

Fig. 1. Similarities in the structures of naloxone, cyclazocine, and naltrexone

naltrexone, had all the desired characteristics. It was like naloxone—a pure narcotic antagonist. In addition, it was partly like cyclazocine, having a long time/action but without the psychotomimetic effects. Once the initial animal studies indicated that naltrexone was not toxic, clinical trials began in 1973. The pharmacodynamic profile of naltrexone in humans was studied in collaboration with Drs. Volavka, Resnick, and Washton of the New York Medical College, and with the collaboration of Drs. Mulé and Kogan in our laboratory (1976).

DISPOSITION OF NALTREXONE

The major metabolite of naltrexone in humans is 6β-naltrexol, isolated by Cone (1973). A minor metabolite, 2-hydroxy-3-methoxy-6β-naltrexol (HMN) was isolated in my laboratory (1975, Fig. 2). The rapid peaking of 6β-naltrexol only an hour after oral administration of naltrexone indicated that a major portion of the drug is biotransformed during its first pass through the liver, converting 75 to 80 percent of the dose to less active metabolites (Fig. 3). The opiate antagonist activity of 6β-naltrexol varies in different species and methods from 1/50th to 1/12th that of naltrexone (Verebey, 1975). Preliminary studies of HMN using the opiate receptor binding assay, prepared from rat synaptosomes, indicated that HMN binding was typically antagonist-like, but its affinity was approximately 1,000 times less than that of naltrexone (Hiller, 1979). Thus the preliminary animal data indicate that among the three compounds naltrexone is the most potent antagonist followed by 6β-naltrexol and the weakest is HMN. However, these relative activities have not been studied in humans.

To determine the major contribution to the narcotic antagonistic effects of naltrexone based not only on potency but also on abundance, the relative concentrations of the three bases were determined in urine, plasma, red blood cells (RBC), and saliva (Verebey, 1980). The patients received 400 mg naltrexone daily, and urine samples were collected 12 hr after the last dose. The relative percentages in urine were 76.6 percent 6β-naltrexol, 14.4 percent HMN, and 9.0 percent naltrexone for the 12-hr spot sample (Table 1). In plasma, collected at the same time as the urine, the relative concentrations were similar: 73.5 percent 6β-naltrexol, 23.1 percent HMN, and 3.4 percent naltrexone (Table 2). It is interesting that no significant amount of 6β-naltrexol was present in RBC and no significant amount of HMN was present in saliva. Even though 6β-naltrexol is less potent than naltrexone, quantitatively it is important and seems to significantly contribute to the narcotic antagonistic activity of the parent compound. HMN, based on the in vitro potency data, appears to be least important.

These observations indicate that individuals who metabolize naltrexone at a slower rate would have longer narcotic antagonism than fast metabolizers. This phenomenon was confirmed by determining the correlation coefficient

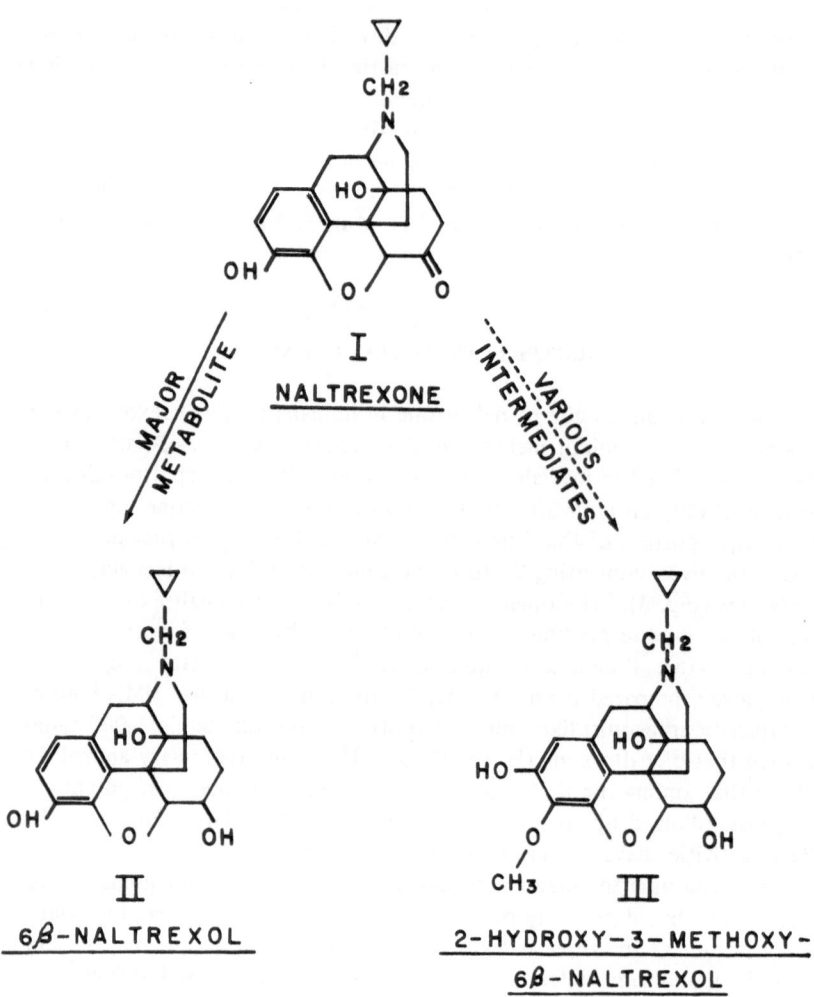

Fig. 2. Major and minor biotransformation pathways of naltrexone in humans

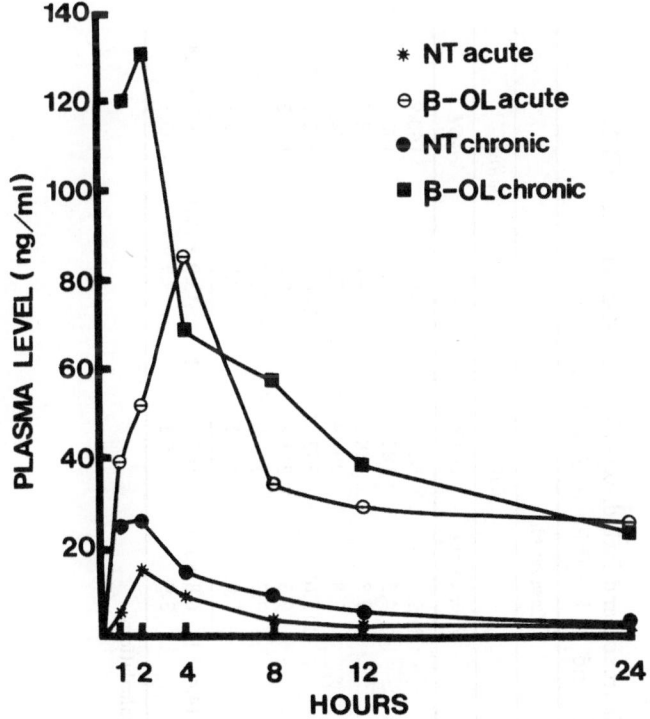

Fig. 3. The plasma levels of naltrexone and 6β-naltrexol after single (acute) and multiple (chronic) doses of 100 mg naltrexone

Table 1.   Urinary Levels of Naltrexone, β-Naltrexol, and 2-Hydroxy-3-Methoxy-6-β-Naltrexol (HMN) in a Single Spot Sample 16 and 24 Hrs After 2X200 mg Naltrexol

| Subject | Base μg/ml | | |
	Naltrexone	β-Naltrexol	HMN
1	10.3	152.0	20.6
1	2.5	62.8	9.1
2	4.5	59.7	12.5
2	5.4	49.4	9.4
3	16.7	131.3	49.7
3	13.9	77.0	49.2
4	43.2	262.3	18.9
4	18.1	184.5	14.6
Mean ± SD	14.3 ± 13.0	122.4 ± 74.8	23.0 ± 16.8
% of total base	8.9	76.7	14.4

Table 2. Plasma and RBC Levels of Naltrexone, β-Naltrexol, and 2-Hydroxy-3-Methoxy-6-β-Naltrexol (HMN) After 2X200 mg Naltrexone Given 24 and 16 Hrs Prior to Sample Collection

Subject	Base ng/ml						
	Plasma			RBC		Saliva	
	Naltrexone	β-Naltrexol	HMN	Naltrexone	HMN	NT	β-OL
1	5.6	143.9	42.7	N.S.	N.S.	20.6	160.9
1	4.8	185.0	55.8	4.3	183.1	4.2	106.7
2	8.7	174.8	74.6	7.3	188.3	4.6	43.5
2	8.2	182.7	65.0	7.8	201.4	7.3	74.0
3	105*	572.2*	151.3*	115.0*	342.6*	246.9*	342.1*
3	10.9	251.8	86.3	9.3	211.8	8.4	151.2
4	20.4	234.2	53.2	7.3	102.0	50.3	571.6
4	6.9	231.5	62.8	5.0	112.5	2.0	59.1
Mean ± SD	9.4 ± 5.2	200.6 ± 39.1	62.9 ± 14.4	6.8 ± 1.9	166.5 ± 47.1	13.9 ± 17.1	166.7 ± 134
% of total base	3.4	73.5	23.1	3.9	96.1	7.7	92.3

*Sample was drawn after naltrexone dose; values not included in the calculations.
N.S. = no samples available.

between individual half-life (t 1/2) values of naltrexone and the responses to heroin challenges 72-hr after the dose in four subjects (Verebey, 1976). The figure indicates that the subject with the longest t 1/2 or slowest metabolizer correlated with the least response to heroin or had the best opiate blockade (Fig. 4).

Another aspect of metabolism which is of concern therapeutically is the possible self-induction of the metabolic rate from an acute dose to chronic drug administration. The relative abundance of 6β-naltrexol and naltrexone was determined in 24-hr urines after acute and chronic administration of naltrexone in four subjects (Table 3). No changes in the ratio (3.31 vs 3.29) indicated no self-induction of naltrexone biotransformation (Verebey, 1976). This is a desirable feature for any drug intended for chronic use because the initial dose remains affective during the whole course of the treatment.

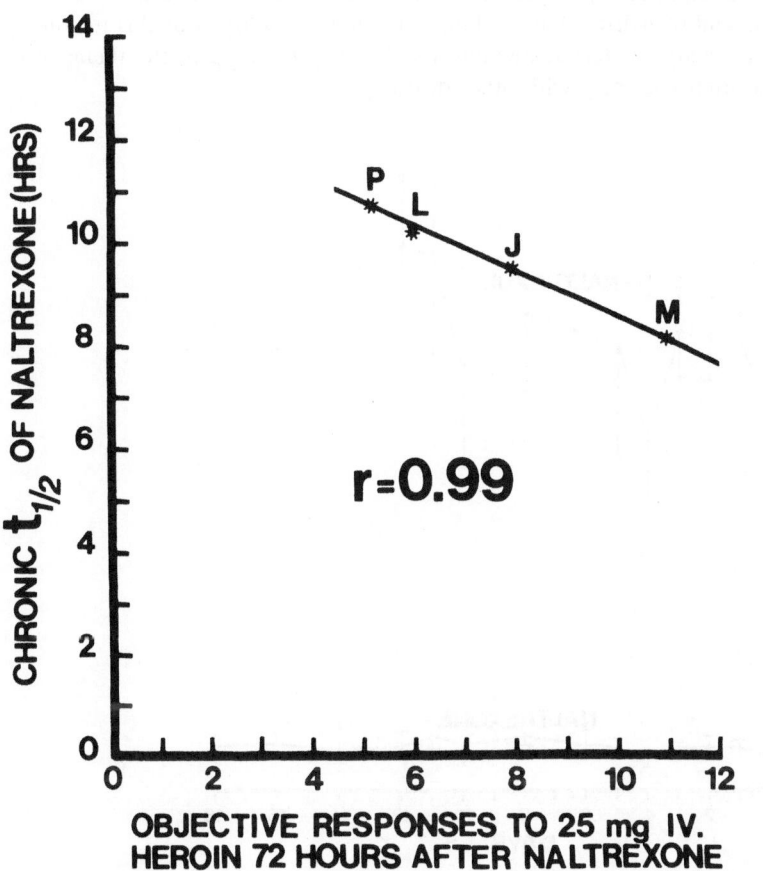

Fig. 4. Correlation between the plasma half-life of naltrexone and the responses to 25 mg IV heroin, 72 hours after naltrexone. Each point represents an individual subject

Table 3. Beta-Naltrexol-Naltrexone Concentration Ratio for the 24-Hr
Urinary Excretion in Acute and Chronic Treatment

	Beta-Naltrexol/Naltrexone	
Subject	Acute	Chronic
C.L.	3.42	2.54
E.M.	3.57	3.96
B.P.	3.55	3.26
R.J.	2.71	3.38
Mean ± SD	3.31 ± 0.41	3.29 ± 0.58

Another indication of the simplicity of naltrexone use in a clinical
setting is the rapid achievement of plasma steady state-equilibrium (Fig. 5).
The figure shows that by the second daily dose, the 24-hr blood levels of
naltrexone and 6β-naltrexol are stabilized (Verebey, 1976). For this reason
it is not necessary to start at low doses and slowly build up to the therapeutic
dose as is often necessary with other drugs.

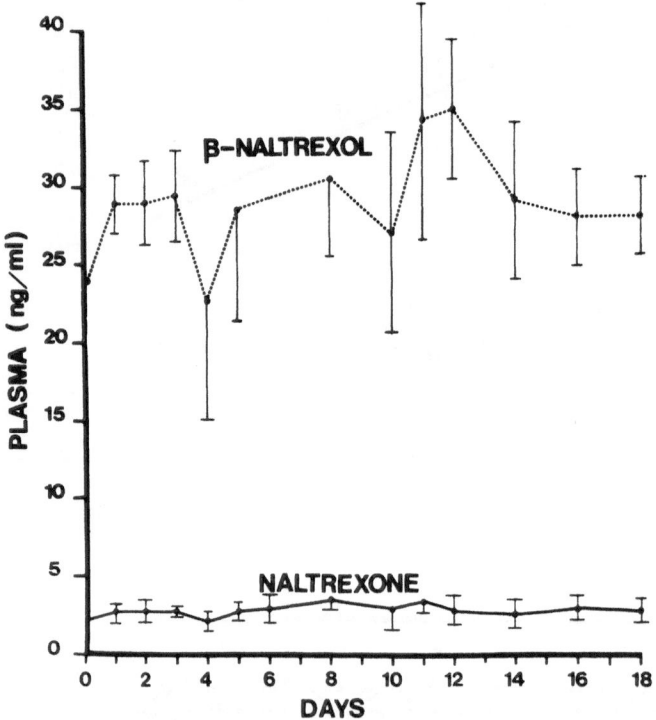

Fig. 5. Naltrexone and 6β-naltrexol plasma levels 24 hours after each daily dose of
100 mg naltrexone

Naltrexone was also studied in schizophrenic patients for its possible use as an antipsychotic drug (Verebey, 1979; Fig. 6). Initial studies failed to indicate promise for that application. However, the rising dose-efficacy study design allowed doses to rise as high as 800 mg/day which are the highest doses ever given to humans. At that dose the average 24-hr plasma level of naltrexone, HMN, and 6β-naltrexol were 9.2, 123, and 331 ng/ml, respectively. There were no signs of toxicity in any of the subjects. Two weeks after the discontinuation of naltrexone the plasma was free of naltrexone and its metabolites indicating very efficient clearance of the drug after chronic administration of large doses (Verebey, 1979).

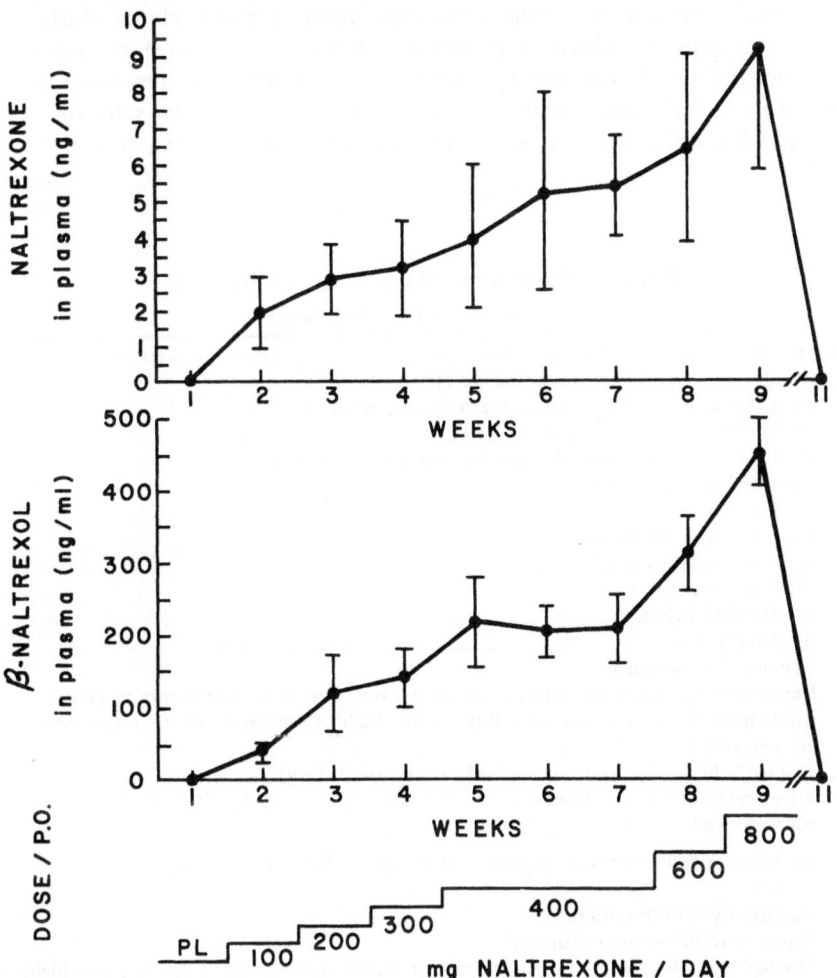

Fig. 6. Naltrexone and 6β-naltrexol plasma levels 24 hours after the designated doses of naltrexone

HEROIN CHALLENGES: THE TIME COURSE OF NARCOTIC BLOCKADE

The opiate receptor blocking activity of naltrexone was studied by challenging it with 25 mg intravenous heroin injections and observing two objective and four subjective responses (Verebey, 1976). A modified version of the Addiction Research Center Inventory was used (Table 4). Opiate symptoms and signs were evaluated separately. The absolute heroin effects were investigated by asking for the ten commonly reported opiate symptoms. The greater number of true responses indicated more complete heroin effects. The relative response was a comparison of the current heroin episode with past heroin experiences. Liking scores represent a state of euphoria which is influenced by the subject's environment. It was scored on a 0 to 4 scale. Another test was devised based on the subject's estimation of how much he would pay for the injection he just received, based on the street value of heroin. The opioid signs constitute measurements and notations of the

Table 4. The Pharmacological Testing Protocols
During and After Heroin Challenges

Opiate Symptoms (reports by the subject about his feelings or physiological state).
1. Absolute—true and false questionnaire (10)
    (a) I feel so good that I know other people can tell it.
    (b) My voice sounds different than usual.
    (c) I feel as if something pleasant has just happened to me.
    (d) I feel it in my stomach.
    (e) I feel it in my mouth.
    (f) I feel it in my throat.
    (g) I feel it in my head.
    (h) I feel it in my nose.
    (i) My skin itches.
    (j) I felt a rush. _____ true
2. Relative—"opiate high"
    Remember the experience when you had the very best high after heroin in your whole life? Now let us say we call it a 100% high. Compared with that, how high are you now? _____ %
3. "Liking" the relative state of euphoria a scale of (0 to 4).
4. Street value of heroin. How much would you pay for this shot if I asked you to pay me now? $ _____

Opiate Signs (measurements or notations of the physiologic state of the subject by observers).
1. Respiratory rate (no./min)
2. Pupillary response (mm diameter)
3. "Liking" the observers' rating of apparent euphoria (no change: 1,2,3,4,5, very high)
4. Pharmacodynamic parameters
    Plasma levels of opiate antagonist at the time of heroin challenge (ng/ml).

subject's physiological state (objective) and the behavioral state (subjective) reported by the observers.

Control heroin related responses were assessed in the absence of naltrexone (Fig. 7). These values were considered 100 percent. During naltrexone treatment using 100 mg daily doses, the narcotic antagonism of naltrexone was challenged by 25 mg heroin injections 24, 48, and 72 hours after the last naltrexone dose. The heroin challenges were at least 10 days apart in the same patient to eliminate the possibility of tolerance development. Observing all test parameters at 24-hr, almost no response was elicited by 25 mg intravenous heroin. However, by 48 and 72-hr after naltrexone some heroin related effects were observed. The overall average responding to

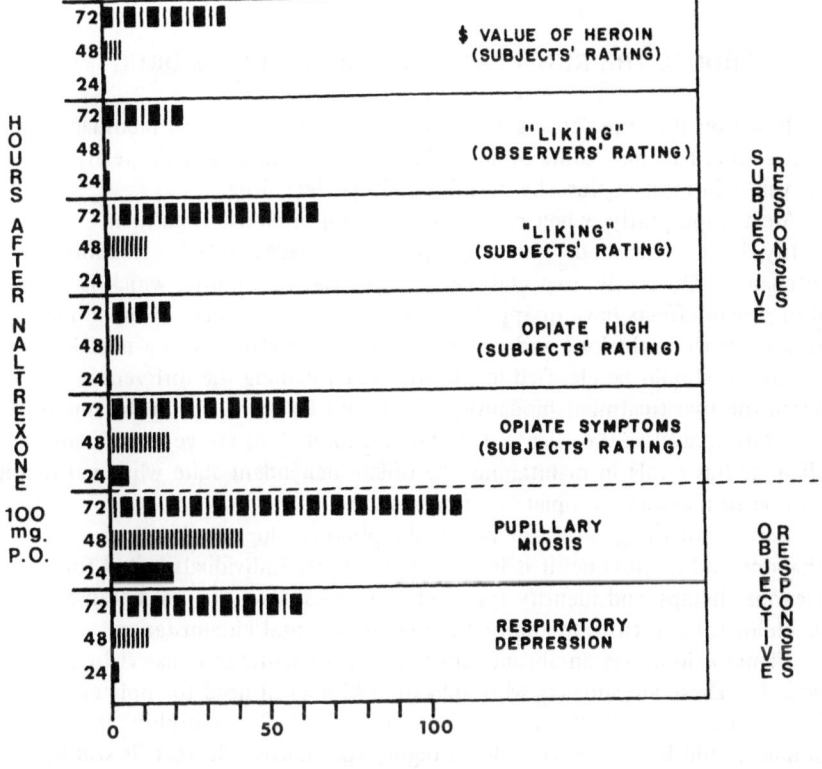

Fig. 7. The percent response to 25 mg heroin 24, 48, and 72 hours after naltrexone of various psychologic and physiologic parameters

heroin were 4.0 percent at 24, 13.5 percent at 48, and 53.4 percent at 72-hr, compared to the 100 percent response in the absence of naltrexone. The subjective heroin related responses were blocked somewhat better and lasted longer. The average subjective responses were 1.2 percent, 8.2 percent, and 42.8 percent for 24, 48, and 72-hr respectively (Verebey, 1976).

It should be emphasized that 25 mg intravenous heroin is a sizable dose, not readily available for most addicts routinely. Thus, the observed length and magnitude of the narcotic blockade seem very effective for most practical preventive measures.

Twenty-four hours after naltrexone the narcotic antagonism was still close to complete yet the blood level of naltrexone is already very low (2.4 ng/ml). The terminal phase plasma level decline is 2.4 to 2.0 to 1.8 ng/ml at 24, 48, and 72-hrs after the last naltrexone dose. This translates into a 98-hr terminal t 1/2 indicating that at 2.4 ng/ml or above complete narcotic antagonism can be maintained (Verebey, 1976).

CHOOSE THE RIGHT PATIENT FOR THE RIGHT DRUG

Based on the experience gained while studying the clinical pharmacology of naltrexone, I formed some opinions in trying to understand the relatively low level of interest in this pharmacologically perfect drug.

Most importantly, when naltrexone first appeared as a treatment modality, it was visualized by most people as a replacement of methadone maintenance. Obviously, expectations of euphoria from a drug which is void of opiate effects have disappointed many early volunteers. Comparing naltrexone with methadone and expecting equivalent effects was a mistake. Expectations should be clarified in the future, explaining the differences between the two treatment modalities. It should be very clear in the minds of the staff as well as the clients that the two modalities are very different. Methadone has a role in maintaining the opiate dependent state while naltrexone has a role to maintain an opiate abstinent state.

Because of the great difference in the pharmacological effects of methadone and naltrexone, it is important to typify individuals suited for naltrexone therapy and identify types who are most likely to fail because of their biological constitution and/or their environmental circumstances.

Figure 8 indicates an abrupt failure point for naltrexone use right below subject A. These are subjects who indicate a biological need for opiates in order to function normally. Before the discovery of the endorphins this reasoning would have been considered highly speculative. In fact, it still has not been proven experimentally that endorphin deficiency or endorphin release problems causes behavioral disturbances which respond to exogenous

OPIATE USE

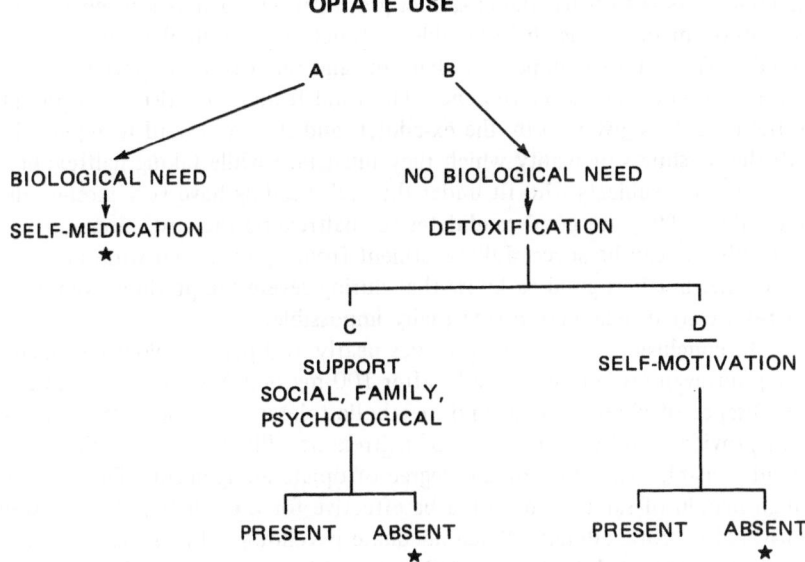

★FAILURE POINTS OF DRUG DETOXIFICATION & NARCOTIC ANTAGONIST
THERAPY

Fig. 8. A proposed model for selection of subjects for successful naltrexone therapy

opioids. The hypothesis that such individuals exist originates from observations made on thousands of methadone maintenance patients during the past
decade. The biological need for opioids is observed especially during
attempted detoxification. A certain percentage of the addict population
when administered less than 15 mg of methadone exhibit acute psychosis,
which is readily reversible by the administration of larger doses of methadone.
Naltrexone blocks all opiate effects; thus a biologically opiate dependent
subject would most likely fail the naltrexone treatment modality regardless
of the external support mechanisms provided.

Most of the addict population, however, is not biologically dependent on
exogenous opioids. This is indicated by the lack of major difficulty during
slow-rate detoxification from methadone. These individuals belong to group
B. Their success with naltrexone therapy requires important supports. The
external support mechanisms are essential at least initially. They consist of
psychological and social counselings and a strong family interest in the subject's fate. Family support is exemplified by a mother, a spouse, or other
family members ascertaining that naltrexone is taken regularly. As long as
naltrexone is taken the subject is in no danger of readdiction. The role of

the counselors is to teach the ex-addict gratifications such as self-reliance and self-improvement, so that he'll be able to function without the crutch of opioids. The external support mechanisms and services are important for the successful clinical use of naltrexone. The total feeling of satisfaction provided by the opioids is given up by the ex-addict, and it is very hard to replace it with the harshness of reality which they must face while taking naltrexone.

The few subjects who fit under the "D" heading have very strong self-motivation. They are good candidates for naltrexone therapy. Some of these subjects can be successfully abstinent from opioids even without naltrexone, but it is good to know that during severe temptations even if opiates are tried, readdiction is virtually impossible.

In conclusion, naltrexone provides nearly 100 percent blockade against 25 mg intravenous heroin for 48-hr after 100 mg oral doses of naltrexone. The absence of pharmacologic and metabolic tolerance during chronic treatment provides carefree clinical use of naltrexone. Plasma level monitoring can provide reliable estimation of the degree of opiate antagonism. The drug has a high margin of safety and should be effective for the rehabilitation of well motivated narcotic addicts. When adequate psychological and social counseling is provided this rehabilitation modality should be very successful.

ACKNOWLEDGEMENTS

Supported by the National Institute on Drug Abuse grant No. DA-01737.

The author thanks Mr. Dennis Jukofsky for proofreading, Mr. Jed Shaw for illustrations and Ms. Reynita Lane for typing the manuscript.

REFERENCES

Blumberg H, Pachter IJ and Matossian Z: US Patent 3, 332, 950 (July 25, 1976)
Cone EJ: Human metabolite of naltrexone (N-cyclopropylmethylnoroxymorphone) with a novel C-6 isomorphine configuration. *Tetrahedron Lett* 23:2607–2610, 1973
Hiller J and Simon E: New York University Medical School, Personal Communication, 1979
Martin WR, Gorodetzky CW and McClane TK: An experimental study in the treatment of narcotic addicts with cyclazocine. *Clin Pharmacol Ther* 7:455–465, 1966
Verebey K and Mulé SJ: Naltrexone pharmacology, pharmacokinetics and metabolism: Current status. *Am J Drug Alcohol Abuse* 2:357–363, 1975
Verebey K and Mulé SJ: Naltrexone and 6β-naltrexol plasma levels in schizophrenic patients after large doses of naltrexone. *Res Commun Psychol, Psychiatry & Behavior* 4:311–317, 1979

Verebey K, Chedekel MA, Mulé SJ and Rosenthal D: Isolation and identification of a new metabolite of naltrexone in human blood and urine. *Res Commun Chem Pathol Pharmacol* 12:67–84, 1975

Verebey K, DePace A, Jukofsky D, Volavka JV and Mulé SJ: Quantitative determination of 2-hydroxy-3-methoxy-6β-naltrexol (HMN), naltrexone, and 6β-naltrexol in human plasma, red blood cells, saliva and urine by gas liquid chromatography. *J Analytical Toxicol* 4:33–37, 1980

Verebey K, Volavka J, Mulé SJ and Resnick RB: Naltrexone: Disposition, metabolism and effects after acute and chronic dosing. *Clin Pharmacol Ther* 20:315–328, 1976

17

Detoxification from Methadone Maintenance: Current and Innovative Approaches

HERBERT D. KLEBER

INTRODUCTION

Detoxification from opiates has created difficulties for as long as these drugs have been available for the relief of pain or the production of euphoria. Although the withdrawal syndrome is rarely life threatening, its symptoms are distressing enough in the acute phase to make it difficult for many addicted individuals to cease use of drugs, and the chronic persistence of low-level symptoms has no doubt been a contributing factor to early relapse. The withdrawal "cures" proposed over the last 100 years have at times been worse than the disease, introducing drugs which are even more addicting or using other methods that either cause more distress or even at times a significant mortality rate. Examples of the former include the use of injectable morphine to cure opium eating (Allbutt, 1870) and the use of heroin to treat morphine addiction (Kramer, 1977); while examples of the latter include the Towns-Lambert belladonna mixture, Narcosan, sodium thiocyanate (Kolb and Himmelsbach, 1938), and electroconvulsive therapy (Thigpen et al, 1953). Because of this distressing history, one must be especially careful in proposing new techniques that they meet the twin demands of safety and efficacy. Any claims for a new method should be put forward with modesty and viewed with skepticism until amply documented by careful experimental procedures.

Approximately 30 years ago, methadone was used in this country to treat the heroin withdrawal syndrome (Isbell and Vogel, 1948) and, approximately 15 years ago, its use was extended to serve as a maintenance agent in treating the narcotic addict (Dole and Nyswander, 1965). In the United

States alone there are currently about 80,000 individuals on methadone maintenance programs, and over 10,000 of these are in the process of withdrawing from methadone at any one time (Senay et al, 1977). While the use of methadone as a withdrawal agent alleviated many of the problems associated with earlier methods of withdrawal, its use as a maintenance agent has created a new set of withdrawal difficulties. The outlook for these 10,000 individuals in the process of withdrawing, and the others to follow, is cloudy. Although figures vary widely from study to study, it can be said as a general rule that no more than 50 percent of the patients attempting detoxification are able to achieve zero dosage at any one time and of those that do, only about 50 percent are able to maintain it (Kleber, 1977). In the classic withdrawal study done by Senay et al (1977), it was found that a slow gradual withdrawal technique over 30 weeks significantly improved the rate obtained compared with detoxification carried out over 10 weeks. Even so, only 53 percent of the patients in the slow withdrawal group were able to achieve zero dosage. Factors such as psychological readiness for withdrawal, age, length of addiction, anxiety, expectation and rate of withdrawal appear to have an important bearing on the outcome (Kissin et al, 1978; Lowinson et al, 1976). Physiological dependence upon methadone may be at least partially responsible for the low rates, but the extent of its role is unclear (Martin et al, 1973). Detoxification becomes more difficult when the dose gets below 20 mg per day (Martin et al, 1977).

Thus, while methadone maintenance, when given in the overall context of a treatment program, has often proven to be a useful tool in aiding the overall rehabilitation of the narcotic addict and his ability to avoid using illicit drugs, patients continue to have a difficult time withdrawing from it even when their social/vocational and psychological situation has changed. Improved detoxification methods would be useful, therefore, in the overall treatment strategy for narcotic addicts. The techniques described below have been tried either for detoxification from heroin, detoxification from methadone, or in both situations.

One important need for improved withdrawal procedures stems from the possibility of switching opiate addicts to the narcotic antagonist, Naltrexone (Martin et al, 1977; Report, 1978). This agent, which blocks the euphoria and addicting potential of narcotics (in appropriate dosages) without being addicting itself can only be used when the individual is off narcotics at least 5-10 days. If taken before this, unpleasant withdrawal symptoms may be precipitated and the patient will drop out of treatment. Using current withdrawal methods which substitute declining doses of methadone for heroin or gradual decrements of the maintained methadone dose, many patients are unable to wait the requisite period drug free and relapse back to opiates

(Resnick et al, 1974). A method which could avoid this drug free wait would increase the usefulness of naltrexone and move treatment closer to the sequence envisioned by Goldstein in his STEPS proposal (Goldstein, 1976).

One must also keep in mind that chronic methadone maintenance might be having untoward effects on endorphin levels and a withdrawal method which enhances the patients' chances for abstinence could decrease the time spent on methadone. Unlike the typical heroin addict on the street whose intake is usually quite variable—high on Monday, sick on Tuesday, less high on Wednesday, etc—the methadone-maintained client is getting a steady dose of a pharmacologically pure and potent medication. This regular intake could lead to suppression of endorphine levels and in some patients the levels might not bounce back even after gradual withdrawal. This should not be taken to mean we should not use methadone. Currently it is the most widely accepted and useful technique for treatment of opiate addicts we have (as long as we remember it is a drug, not a treatment, and must be given in a context of psychosocial supports and therapy) (Kleber, 1980). As clinicians, therefore, we need it for our patients. As scientists, however, we must continue to point out potential flaws, risks, etc, in any method we use and continue to strive for better ones. Finally, in this context, one must add that the long-term effect of naltrexone on possible endorphin suppression is also not known.

PROPANOLOL

Propanolol, a beta-adrenergic blocking agent, has been tried in the treatment of narcotic withdrawal. It was found that patients treated with the drug required a somewhat smaller methadone dose for detoxification and that the patients who responded favorably had milder withdrawal symptoms. The overall conclusion, however, was the "the small benefit from the drug hardly merits its consideration as an adjunct to the treatment of withdrawal from opiates" (Hollister and Prusmack, 1974).

The attempt to use propanolol in narcotic withdrawal was suggested by the work of Grosz (1972) who noted that propanolol given to heroin addicts abolished the euphoric effect of the narcotic as well as the compulsive craving for the opiate which followed heroin withdrawal. Although he did not feel that the drug helped in the management of the acute physical withdrawal syndrome, Hollister et al (Hollister and Prusmack, 1974), decided to try it anyway because Grosz had noted that it possessed narcotic antagonist potential.

PROPOXYPHENE

Propoxyphene, a mild analgesic derived from methadone but having less addictive and analgesic potential, has been tried to relieve the symptoms of narcotic withdrawal, and particularly its napsylate form has received a good deal of attention in this regard. The napsylate form is only slightly soluble in water, whereas propoxyphene hydrochloride is very water soluble. This lowered water solubility leads to slower absorption in the g.i. tract, lower peak plasma levels, and, therefore, it is believed to have a much lower overdose potential. Because of the similarities to methadone and because, at times, it has been difficult to use methadone in many places on an out-patient basis for withdrawal, programs have tried the propoxyphene napsylate for withdrawal. The results to date suggest that while this drug is not as good an agent as methadone in suppressing the full spectrum of narcotic withdrawal, it can partially block the development of withdrawal symptoms with the notable exception of insomnia (Tennant, 1974; Inaba et al, 1974). Because it is addicting itself and because, especially mixed with alcohol, the additive effects on respiratory depression can be fatal, it is important that, if the drug be used, the amounts given the patient to take by prescription be not excessive. The studies seemed to indicate that 800–1,000 mg a day given in two or three divided doses is sufficient. It should also be pointed out that this use of propoxyphene in either the hydrochloride or napsylate form is not an approved indication for the drugs and that, if research is to be done, an IND would be required from the Food and Drug Administration. Since October 1980 it has been illegal to use it for withdrawal without an IND from the FDA.

ACUPUNCTURE

The use of acupuncture to manage pain goes back thousands of years in Chinese medicine. Its use to treat narcotic withdrawal is a relatively recent phenomena, however, with the first paper reporting results in 1973 by Wen and Cheung (1973). They report on 40 patients using acupuncture with electrical stimulation. This paper as well as others, were critically reviewed by Whitehead (1978), who concluded that, "the use of acupuncture in the management of withdrawal symptoms is insufficiently reported as to constitute an adequate clinical trial. No control subjects and no control conditions have been employed. Those results that have been reported are incomplete and inadequate and these same results have been misinterpreted by others in the direction of 'gilding the lily' . . . " In later papers, Chen (1977) suggested that acupuncture may work by stimulating enkephalin in release, and Wen (1977) reported that if patients were treated with naloxone at the same time as receiving acupuncture, the whole procedure was markedly shortened.

Although a controlled trial would add considerably to evaluation of the technique, there is debate over the possibility of a double-blind trial. Even without this, it appears that acupuncture with electrical stimulation (AES) has some effect on withdrawal symptoms but is cumbersome, has to be given frequently, and takes seven to eight days to detoxify patients. The new procedure using naloxone may improve the usefulness of the technique but better designed studies need to be done to prove this.

VITAMIN C

Since high doses of ascorbic acid (vitamin C) have been used to treat or prevent a number of conditions as varied as the common cold, heart disease, leprosy, and viral hepatitis, it is not surprising that it would be tried with narcotic withdrawal. Libby and Stone (1977) reported 100 cases of heroin addicts they had detoxified using doses of ascorbic acid in the 25–85 mg/day range. The patients were treated for one to two weeks in a residential setting and then discharged on holding doses of 10 gram/day. The patients reported a loss of craving for narcotics while taking the mega-doses of vitamin C. Free and Sanders (1978) reported an outpatient trial of the ascorbic acid regime. Patients volunteered for one of three groups—ascorbic acid only, symptomatic medications (eg, propoxyphene, librium, chlorahydrate), and symptomatic medications for three days followed by mega-dose ascorbic acid. Group 1 had 30 clients, Group 2 had 186 clients and Group 3 had 11 clients. The combined group reported fewer withdrawal symptoms and a shorter withdrawal period. In addition, many subjects in either Group 1 or 3 using ascorbic acid reported increased energy, loss of drug craving and some block of narcotic effect if they used narcotics while they were taking the vitamin C. Doses of vitamin C in Group 1 were 24–48 g/day for five to seven days, tapering to 8–12 g/day for 14 days. In addition to the vitamin C, patients were given multivitamin amd mineral preparations, calcium and magnesium tablets, and liquid protein.

Although no side effects other than nausea in one subject and a rash in a second one were reported, mega-doses of vitamin C have been suggested to cause kidney stones, destruction of vitamin B_{12}, pentosuria, and possible increased chance of infertility and abortion. Given these possible complications, the fact that the two trials to date were uncontrolled studies, and that the improvement noted was not very large, mega-dose ascorbic acid treatment should be considered experimental and risky.

NALOXONE PRECIPITATED WITHDRAWAL

Although the usual methods of withdrawal tend toward the slow gradual approach, some authors have tried to markedly compress the abstinence syndrome on the theory that total discomfort may be less in such an approach even though the peak may be higher. Both Blatchly et al (1975) and Resnick et al (1975) have used naloxone-precipitated withdrawal to bring about this shortened detoxification syndrome. The technique consists primarily of giving i.m., or i.v. naloxone repeatedly at frequent intervals for one or two days until further injections produce no withdrawal symptoms. Blatchly used dioperidol, propanolol, and Ketamine to handle the symptoms produced but these agents had minimal ameliorating effect. Resnick initially used amobarbital, atropine and chlorpromazine but later gave nothing except nighttime sedation and found the acute symptoms subsided about an hour after each dose. More recently he has premedicated with diazepam and atropine (Resnick et al, 1977). Probably because of the persistence of unpleasant symptoms, the technique has not caught on and is rarely used.

CLONIDINE

Gold, Redmond, and Kleber first reported in 1978 (Gold et al, 1978) that clonidine, an alpha adrenergic agonist used to treat hypertension, could suppress or reverse the symptoms of opiate withdrawal. They have since published a number of papers on this (Gold et al, 1978; 1979a; 1979b; 1980), extending the original findings and their results have been confirmed by Washton and Resnick (1979). The major withdrawal symptoms not totally blocked are insomnia and irritability. Clonidine has been used to treat both heroin and methadone withdrawal. The usual regime for methadone with-drawal from doses of up to 25 mg methadone/day (in an individual of average weight—approximately 70–75 Kg) is as follows:

Day 1   —0.1 mg clonidine test dose in a.m.
          0.2 mg at 5 p.m.
          0.2 mg at 10 p.m.
Day 2   —0.2 mg three times a day
Day 3–10 —0.3 mg three times a day (may vary between total dose of
          0.8–1.5)
Day 11   —half of dose of Day 10
Day 12   —half of dose of Day 11
Day 13   —half of dose of Day 12

For heroin withdrawal, the length of the clonidine treatment can usually be reduced to four days and lower doses can be used. To check for completeness of detoxification, a naloxone test dose (0.8 mgm) can be given the next day to see if any symptoms are precipitated.

The major side-effects of clonidine are sedation and lowered blood pressure so patients should be checked for this up to two hours after each dose. If blood pressure is less than 85/60 at the time to receive the next clonidine dose, it should be postponed until the pressure has risen. There have also been instances of acute psychiatric problems after clonidine detoxification is over so patients with a prior history of schizophrenia or major affective disorder should probably be excluded from this technique. It is important to keep in mind that although clonidine increases the chance of an individual completing detoxification, it does nothing to keep addict off and the relapse rate remains at 50 percent or higher.

The total daily dose of clonidine may need to be less on an outpatient than inpatient regime because of the problems of sedation and hypotension. On an outpatient basis, patients should be warned about the sedative effects of clonidine especially in relation to driving and operating machinery. Patients probably should not drive at least the first five days of being on the drug and longer if sedation or hypotension is a problem. To deal with persistent insomnia, one should use sedatives such as chloral hydrate. Patients should be warned that mixing alcohol with the clonidine can be especially dangerous because of alcohol's hypotensive effect. Amitriptyline if started after clonidine, may also increase the hypotensive effect.

The discovery of clonidine's acting on opiate withdrawal has suggested the following model of how withdrawal takes place in the brain.

" . . . opiate withdrawal may be due, in part, to increased noradrenergic neural activity in areas such as the locus coeruleus which are regulated by both opiates through opiate receptors and clonidine through alpha-2 adrenergic receptors. . . . Opiates administered systemically turn off the locus coeruleus by stimulation of inhibitory opiate receptor sites with reversal of this effect by the opiate antagonist, naloxone. Clonidine also inhibits the locus coeruleus but by stimulation of a different receptor, this effect being reversed by specific alpha-2 adrenergic antagonists . . . " (Gold et al, 1980).

CLONIDINE-NALOXONE

Building on the naloxone flush technique of Resnick et al (1975) and Blachly et al (1975) and the clonidine work of Gold, Redmond and Kleber (1978), Riordan and Kleber (1980a; 1980b) combined the two techniques to produce an ultra short and yet comfortable method of withdrawal. Patients on doses up to 30 mg/day of methadone have their dose abruptly halted and are given clonidine 0.7 mg in divided doses on day 1. On day 2 this is increased to 1.2 mg in divided doses and Naloxone i.v. or i.m. is given hourly in increasing doses.

Typically: 8:00 a.m.–clonidine 0.4 mg and at 2 + hours

9:30 a.m.–Naloxone 0.1

10:30 a.m.–Naloxone 0.1

11:30 a.m.–Naloxone 0.2

Day 2:   12:30 p.m.–Naloxone 0.2

1:30 p.m.–Naloxone 0.3

2:30 p.m.–Naloxone 0.3

3:30 p.m.–Naloxone 0.4 X 4 doses

on

8:00 a.m.–Clonidine 0.4 and at 2 p.m.

9:30 a.m.–Naloxone 0.4

10:30 a.m.–Naloxone 0.4

Day 3:   11:30 a.m.–Naloxone 0.4

12:30 p.m.–Naloxone 0.4

1:30 p.m.–Naloxone 0.8 X 6 doses

Chloral hydrate 1 Gm is given as needed for sleep. On day 4 1.2 mg Naloxone is given as test dose. We have also noted that on day 6 some discomfort occurs and is relieved by low doses clonidine 0.1 b.i.d. for a few days. We hypothesize that using naltrexone from day 4 on may prevent these mild withdrawal symptoms. We are currently trying to modify the technique so it can be done all orally using naltrexone instead of naloxone with an eye to possible outpatient use.

ISBELL/WIKLER 1948 STUDIES

Before closing it may be useful to be reminded of what it is we are trying to treat. Current studies indicate it is especially hard to get from 25–30 mg/day of methadone to zero whereas going from the higher doses to 25 mg is not that difficult. Most attrition occurs at the lower dosage and may relate to methadone at those doses not lasting a full 24 hours so patients have daily withdrawal symptoms. When Isbell and Vogell studied methadone in 1948, they addicted individuals to doses as high as 200–400 mg/day and then abruptly stopped all medication. Their results were as follows:

Changes Following Withdrawal of Methadone

Withdrawal of methadone was abrupt and complete in all cases. Observations were carried out for only six days on the ten men who received the drug for twenty-eight to fifty-six days. The

six-day period of observation was based on experience with the
morphine abstinence syndrome and is sufficiently long for
evaluating the withdrawal sickness after discontinuance of the
use of morphine. However, because of the continuation of
complaints by these 10 subjects, who were the first from whom
methadone was withheld, after discharge from the research ward,
the observation period was extended to fourteen days for the five
men who were given doses producing addiction for four and a half
to six months.

   After withdrawal, a definite abstinence syndrome ensued in
all fifteen cases. The manifestations of this syndrome, though
milder than those seen after the withdrawal of morphine, were
consistently observed in all men and at the same time. Subjectively,
the men made no complaints in the first two days of abstinence
and said that they were still under the influence of the drug (were
"loaded"). On the third day of abstinence they began to complain
of anxiety, insomnia, vague gastric distress, headache and occasionally, tinnitus. The men did not suffer from the muscle
aches and cramps which are so troublesome after the withdrawal
of morphine. The subjective symptoms increased in intensity
until the sixth day of abstinence, after which they gradually
declined. Some patients continued to complain of weakness for
sixty days after withdrawal. Thirteen of the fifteen subjects
considered the subjective symptoms less severe than those following
the abrupt withdrawal of morphine, but all agreed that the symptoms
were sufficiently severe to cause them to return to the use of the
drug had it been obtainable. Nearly all complained bitterly about
the slowness in improvement. A typical comment on the tenth
day of abstinence was 'This stuff seems like it never will turn a
man loose. When I stop a morphine habit I start getting better on
the third day and keep getting better every day after that. I
didn't start to get sick until the third day off, and I'm still half
sick all the time and not getting better. If I were on the street
I'd have a shot within five minutes.'

   The general appearance and behavior of fourteen of the men
were not greatly altered. They appeared to be tired and mildly
irritable. They made frequent requests for either methadone or
morphine after the third day of abstinence but did not lose
emotional control when their requests were refused" (Isbell et al,
1948)

CONCLUSION

   Narcotic addiction is both a psycho-social and physiological condition.
The high percentage of Vietnam veterans addicted to heroin while in Vietnam

who were *not* addicted a year later when back in the United States, as well as the overwhelming majority of medically addicted individuals who cease narcotic use once the underlying painful condition is treated, all bear witness to the important role of psychological and social factors. Conversely, the existence of the opiate receptor sites, the endorphins, and the protracted abstinence syndrome, are significant reminders of the potential role which biological factors play. Our clinical experience with clonidine to date supports the necessity of adequate psychological supports during and after the withdrawal process. The patients in many cases have been on a daily drug, whether heroin or methadone, for 5 to 15 years. Sudden cessation of this daily drug intake, around which many of their daily activities were scheduled, is often felt as an acute loss or disorienting factor with resultant depression, confusion, and, finally, return to drug use. We have learned through painful experience that during clonidine administration, patients should have a daily opportunity to talk about what they are going through with a knowledgeable clinician, and they should remain in treatment afterwards for at least one to three months. Where the size of the program permits, it may be useful to establish a clonidine group where patients who have undergone clonidine-aided withdrawal can meet at least once a week and discuss with a skilled group leader the problems involved in remaining abstinent and the experiential psychological loss. Although this support can be crucial, it is too often spurned by patients who feel that once they are clean they wish no further program contact.

REFERENCES

Allbutt C: On the abuse of hypodermic injections of morphine. *Practitioner* 3:327, 1870

Blachly RH, Casey D, Marcel L and Denney DD: Rapid detoxification from heroin and methadone maintenance using naloxone. A model for study of the treatment of the opiate abstinence syndrome. In: Senay E, Shorty V and Alkesne H (eds) *Developments in the Field of Drug Abuse.* Cambridge, Massachusetts, 1975

Chen GS: Enkephalin, drug addiction and acupuncture. *Amer J Chinese Med* 5:25-30, 1977

Dole VP and Nyswander M: A medical treatment for diacetylmorphine (heroin) addiction. *JAMA* 193:646-650, 1965

Free V and Sanders P: The use of ascorbic acid and mineral supplements in the detoxification of narcotic addicts. *J Orthomolecular Psychiatry* 7:264-270, 1978

Gold MS, Pottash ALC, Sweeney DR and Kleber HD: Clonidine: A safe, effective and rapid non-opiate treatment for opiate withdrawal. *JAMA* 243:343-346, 1980

Gold MS, Pottash ALC, Sweeney DR and Kleber HD: Rapid opiate detoxification: Clinical evidence of antidepressant and antipanic effects of opiates. *Amer J Psychiatry* 136:982-983, 1979b

Gold MS, Pottash ALC, Sweeney DR and Kleber HD: The effect of methadone dosage on clonidine detoxification efficacy. *Amer J Psychiatry* 137:375-376, 1980

Gold MS, Redmond DE and Kleber HD: Clonidine blocks acute opiate withdrawal symptoms. *Lancet* 2:599–602, 1978

Gold MS, Redmond DE and Kleber HD: Clonidine in opiate withdrawal. *Lancet* 1: 929–930, 1978

Gold MS, Redmond DE and Kleber HD: Noradrenergic hyperactivity in opiate withdrawal supported by clonidine reversal of opiate withdrawal. *Amer J Psychiatry* 136: 100–102, 1979

Goldstein A: Heroin addiction: Sequential treatment employing pharmacologic supports. *Arch Gen Psychiatry* 33:353–358, 1976

Grosz HJ: Narcotic withdrawal symptoms in heroin users treated with propanolol. *Lancet* 2:564–566, 1972

Hollister LE and Prusmack JJ: Propanolol in withdrawal from opiates. *Arch Gen Psychiatry* 31:695–698, 1974

Inaba DS, Mewmeyer JA, Gay GR and Whitehead CA: I got a yen for that darvon N: A pilot study on the use of propoxyphene napsylate in the treatment of heroin addiction. *Amer J Drug Alcohol Use* 1:67–78, 1974

Isbell H and Vogel VH: The addiction liability of methadone and its use in the treatment of the morphine abstinence syndrome. *Amer J Psychiatry* 105:909–914, 1948

Isbell H, Wikler A, Eisenman AM, Daingerfield M and Frank K: Liability of addiction to 6-dimethylamino-4-4-diphenyl-3-heptanone (methadone, 'amidone,' or '10820') in man. *Arch Int Med* 81:362–392, 1948

Kissin B, Arnon D and Luckom-Nurnberg F: Patient acceptability and clinical applicability of alternative treatment methods. *New York Acad Sci* 311:282–295, 1978

Kleber HD: Detoxification from methadone maintenance: The state of the art. *Int J Addict* 12(7):807–820, 1977

Kleber HD: Methadone maintenance: Problems and perspectives. *Psychiatry Letter*, submitted for publication.

Kolb L and Himmelsbach CK: Clinical studies of drug addiction. III. A critical review of the withdrawal treatments with method of evaluating abstinence syndromes. *Public Health Reports* 128:1–33, 1938

Kramer JC: Heroin in the treatment of morphine addiction. *J Psychedelic Drugs* 9(3):193–197, 1977

Libby A and Stone I: The hypoascorbemia-kwaskiorkor approach to drug addiction therapy: A pilot study. *J Orthomolecular Psychiatry* 6:300–308, 1977

Lowinson J, Berle B and Longrod J: Detoxification of long-term methadone patients: Problems and prospects. *Int J Addict* 11(6):1009–1013, 1976

Martin WR, Jasinsky DR, Haertzen CA and Kay DC: Methadone—A re-evaluation. *Arch Gen Psychiatry* 23:286–295, 1973

Martin WR, Jasinski DR and Mansky RA: Naltrexone, an antagonist for treatment of heroin dependence. *Arch Gen Psychiatry* 28:784–791, 1977

Report of the National Research Council Committee on Clinical Evaluation of Narcotic Antagonists: Clinical evaluation of naltrexone treatment of opiate-dependence individuals. *Arch Gen Psychiatry* 35:335–340, 1978

Resnick RB, Kestenbaum RS, Washton A and Poole D: Naloxone-precipitated withdrawal: A method for rapid induction onto naltrexone. *Clin Pharmac Therap* 21:409–413, 1977

Resnick R, Kestenbaum R, Gaztanaga P, Volavka J and Freedman AM: Experimental techniques for rapid withdrawal from methadone maintenance: Results of pilot trials. In: Senay E, Shorty V and Alkesne H (eds) *Developments in the Field of Drug Abuse*. Cambridge, Massachusetts, 1975

Resnick RB, Volavka J, Freedman AH and Thomas M: Studies on EN 1639A
    (naltrexone): A new narcotic antagonist. *Amer J Psychiatry* 131:646–650, 1974
Riordan CE and Kleber HD: Clonidine-naloxone approach to methadone withdrawal.
    Submitted for publication, 1980b
Riordan CE and Kleber HD: Rapid opiate detoxification with clonidine and naloxone.
    Lancet 1(8187):1079–1080, 1980a
Senay EC, Dorus W, Goldberg F and Thorton W: Withdrawal from methadone
    maintenance. *Arch Gen Psychiatry* 34:361–367, 1977
Senay EC, Dorus W, Goldberg F and Thorton W: Withdrawal from methadone main-
    tenance: Rate of withdrawal and expectation. *Services Research Report* N.I.D.A.:
    1–19, 1977
Tennant FS: Propoxyphene napsylate for heroin addiction. *JAMA* 266:1212–1214, 1974
Tennant FS, Russell BA, Casas SK and Bleich RN: Heroin detoxification—A comparison
    of propoxyphene and methadone. *JAMA* 232:1019–1022, 1975
Thigpen FB, Thigpen CH and Cleckley HM: Use of electric-convulsive therapy in
    morphine, meperidine, and related alkaloid addictions. *Arch Neurol Psychiatry*
    70:452–458, 1953
Washton AM, Resnick RB and Rossen A: Clonidine hydrochloride: A non-opiate
    treatment for opiate withdrawal. Proceedings of the 41st Annual Scientific
    Meeting of the Committee on Problems of Drug Dependence. National
    Institute on Drug Abuse. Monograph, 1979
Wen HL: Fast detoxification of heroin addicts by acupuncture and electrical stimulation
    (AES) in combination with naloxone. *Comp Med East West* 5:257–263, 1977
Wen HL and Cheung SYC: Treatment of drug addiction by acupuncture and electrical
    stimulation. *Amer J Acupuncture* 1:71–75, 1973
Whitehead PC: Acupuncture in the treatment of addiction: A review and analysis.
    Int J Addict 13:1–16, 1978

18

Clonidine and Lofexidine: New Nonopiate Treatments for Opiate Withdrawal

ARNOLD M. WASHTON
RICHARD B. RESNICK

INTRODUCTION

Recent studies (Gold et al, 1978; Washton et al, 1980a) showing that the non-opiate antihypertensive agent, clonidine hydrochloride, suppresses signs and symptoms of opiate withdrawal, have suggested that clonidine and similar drugs might be useful in the clinical management of opiate detoxification. The fact that clonidine is not an opiate drug and does not itself produce addiction or euphoria suggests some unique and potentially useful applications of this medication in the treatment of opiate-dependent persons. For example, clonidine might be used to block the emergence of abstinence symptoms during a gradual methadone detoxification. Clonidine might also serve as a transitional treatment between opiate dependence and induction onto the long-acting opiate antagonist, naltrexone (Resnick et al, 1979). If withdrawal symptoms were controlled by clonidine, patients might be able to abruptly discontinue chronic opiate use and remain abstinent during the minimum 10-day opiate-free period that is required before starting naltrexone aftercare treatment. In general, clonidine might increase the chances of detoxification success and allow patients greater access to naltrexone and drug-free modalities.

Since the initial report (Gold et al, 1978) of clonidine's withdrawal-suppressing effects in opiate addicts, a variety of clinical studies have explored the usefulness of this medication in opiate detoxification, as reviewed recently by Washton and Resnick (1981). The present chapter describes the out-patient studies conducted at New York Medical College with patients addicted to heroin and/or methadone. Also described is recent work with lofexidine, an analogue of clonidine that appears to be a safer and more effective non-opiate treatment for opiate withdrawal.

CLONIDINE

Our first study (Washton et al, 1980a) sought to replicate the single-dose findings of Gold et al (1978) in order to gather additional information on the physiological and subjective effects of clonidine in opiate-dependent humans. A single oral dose of 0.2 or 0.3 mg clonidine was administered to 12 opiate-dependent outpatients experiencing acute withdrawal from heroin and/or methadone. Blood pressure and ratings for the presence and severity of withdrawal symptoms were taken immediately before clonidine administration and at 2 hours postclonidine. The data showed that clonidine produced a marked and significant reduction in subjective withdrawal severity. The particular symptoms reduced most effectively by clonidine were chills, lacrimation, rhinorrhea, yawning, stomach cramps, sweating, and muscle and joint aches. Marked reductions in anxiety and restlessness were also reported. Side effects were dry mouth, drowsiness, and a decrease of 10–15 mmHg in systolic and diastolic blood pressure. None of the 12 subjects experienced euphoria or any other opiate-like effects from clonidine, and none reported unpleasant side effects.

We subsequently explored clonidine's usefulness as an adjunct to methadone dose reductions and also as a transitional treatment during the 10-day period between opiate dependence and naltrexone. In an initial outpatient trial (Washton and Resnick, 1980a) with 20 methadone-dependent volunteers, an attempt was made to determine whether clonidine could be used to prevent emergence of abstinence symptoms during the course of gradual methadone dose reductions. This study addressed the issue of prophylactic blockade of the abstinence syndrome in contrast to the previous studies (Gold et al, 1978; Washton et al, 1980a) that used clonidine to reduce ongoing withdrawal symptoms. Patients taking 10–50 mg methadone daily were inducted onto clonidine doses of 0.5–0.9 mg per day before initiating methadone dose reductions of 5 or 10 mg per week. All patients had been taking clonidine for at least two weeks before the methadone detoxification was begun. Ten of the 20 patients (50 percent) reached a zero methadone dose and remained opiate-free on clonidine for 10 days before starting naltrexone. Although the patients who successfully completed the detoxification generally complained of less severe and fewer symptoms than the patients who failed, it was evident that clonidine did not totally prevent the emergence of withdrawal symptoms. Patients who complained of intense withdrawal discomfort tended to be those who had been taking clonidine for more than three weeks, suggesting the development of tolerance to clonidine's antiwithdrawal effects.

In another outpatient trial (Washton et al, 1980b), clonidine was administered to 88 opiate-dependent volunteers following abrupt discontinuation of methadone or heroin. Forty-three patients had received methadone 5–40 mg daily (mean 15 mg), and the other 45 patients had been taking illicit methadone or heroin in varying doses. On day 1, all patients received placebo methadone and started a self-administered clonidine dose regimen of 0.1 mg qid with gradual increases as needed over succeeding days. The maximum daily clonidine dose averaged 0.8 mg (range 0.3–1.2 mg). On day 10, patients who showed opiate-free urines and denied using any illicit opiates while on clonidine were given a naloxone challenge of 2.0 mg IV to assess their readiness to begin treatment with naltrexone. Seventy-two percent of the 43 methadone maintenance patients and 50 percent of illicit opiate users completed detoxification and started naltrexone treatment. Those who were on the higher doses of heroin and/or methadone had the greatest difficulty in completing detoxification. All patients reported that clonidine reduced, but did not eliminate their withdrawal discomfort. Lethargy and insomnia were the most frequent and persistent residual complaints. Most patients experienced some mild dizziness or lightheadedness upon standing, but these side effects were unacceptably severe in only six cases. No single clonidine dose regimen was best for all patients, because sensitivity to clonidine's effects varied widely among individuals. To achieve effective control of withdrawal symptoms without untoward side effects, it was necessary to individualize the clonidine dose regimen according to each patient's blood pressure and symptomatology.

Rawson et al (1981) provided additional evidence of clonidine's effectiveness in outpatient opiate withdrawal and found that the availability of naltrexone aftercare treatment significantly increased detoxification success rates. Among patients offered clonidine as a transitional treatment between methadone and naltrexone, nine of 12 (75 percent) achieved 10 days of opiate abstinence and started naltrexone, whereas only three of 12 (25 percent) in a group offered clonidine but no naltrexone achieved 10 days abstinence. The differential efficacy of the clonidine detoxification procedure between the two groups of subjects did not appear to result from differences in the degree to symptom relief, but rather from different subject attitudes toward their detoxification. Subjects in the clonidine/naltrexone group perceived the clonidine detoxification as a transitional treatment with a specific goal. Naltrexone induction on day 10 postmethadone was perceived as a clear endpoint to the detoxification. Subjects in this group frequently expressed the feeling that they had "made it" when they started naltrexone and many reported feeling relief that once on naltrexone they no longer had to struggle with the urges and cravings to use opiates. It appeared that if the clonidine procedure was perceived by subjects as being for a specific number of days with a clear goal and endpoint such as starting naltrexone, most of them could exert sufficient control to abstain from opiate use for the 10 days postmethadone. Subjects in the clonidine-only group did not view the detoxification process as having a clear endpoint or goal and this seemed to contribute to their inability to resist opiate cravings.

Although the clinical studies summarized above were encouraging, none compared clonidine against other detoxification methods. We recently reported a double-blind outpatient study (Washton and Resnick, 1980b) in which 26 volunteers dependent on methadone (15–30 mg daily) were randomly assigned to a clonidine or methadone detoxification procedure. The clonidine procedure (N=13) consisted of abrupt substitution of clonidine for methadone on day 1 of the study. The methadone procedure (N=13) consisted of methadone dose reductions of 1 mg per day until a zero dose was reached. Both procedures were placebo controlled with daily regimens of active or placebo clonidine tablets individualized by a physician who was not aware of the patient's assigned treatment group. No significant difference was found between the clonidine and methadone procedures in terms of the numbers of patients who completed a 10-day opiate-abstinence period after the last dose of active methadone. Four of 13 subjects (38 percent) were successful with clonidine, and six of 13 (46 percent) were successful with methadone (p > 0.05, chi-square test). Major withdrawal symptoms were nearly identical for both groups and consisted mainly of lethargy, restlessness, and insomnia. The clinical course of subjects was distinctly different for the clonidine and methadone procedures, making it impossible to maintain truly double-blind conditions. Subjects taking clonidine reported sedation, dry mouth, occasional dizziness, and onset of withdrawal symptoms within the first 2–3 days of the study. By contrast, subjects taking methadone reported no sedation, dry mouth, or dizziness, and no major withdrawal symptoms until the final week of the procedure when methadone doses were approaching zero milligrams.

LOFEXIDINE

Clonidine's efficacy in suppressing opiate withdrawal has suggested that other alpha-2 noradrenergic agonists might also be effective in opiate with-drawal but without untoward side effects. Lofexidine is an investigational analogue of clonidine that has been shown to suppress opiate withdrawal in morphine-dependent rats (Shearman et al, 1980). Clinical testing in human hypertensive patients (Maner et al, 1980; St. John LaCorte et al, 1981) has suggested that lofexidine's sedative and hypotensive effects are less potent than those of clonidine.

We have recently completed an open clinical trial of lofexidine in opiate detoxification (Washton et al, 1981). As in our earlier studies with

clonidine, the clinical test of lofexidine's usefulness was conducted in an outpatient setting with the measure of detoxification success defined by induction
onto naltrexone. Our subjects were fifteen methadone-dependent male outpatient volunteers who showed no evidence of medical or psychiatric illness
and gave informed consent to the study which involved an abrupt switch from
methadone to lofexidine. On day 1, subjects received their usual methadone
dose (10–25 mg) and began a self-administered lofexidine dose regimen of
0.1 mg two or three times daily. On day 2, methadone was abruptly discontinued with subjects receiving a matched placebo methadone solution and
the lofexidine dosage was increased to 0.1 mg four times daily. Subsequently,
the lofexidine dose was increased as needed to no more than 0.4 mg four times
daily according to symptoms and side effects. All subjects were told that the
detoxification procedure would take 11 days and that naltrexone could be
started on day 11 (10 days postmethadone) provided that they used no
illicit opiates during the study as confirmed by the absence of a precipitated
withdrawal reaction to intravenous naloxone challenge (2.0 mg) on day 11.
Subjects who did use illicit opiates during the first 10 days postmethadone
were allowed to continue on lofexidine and the naloxone challenge was
postponed to the first opportunity where it posed minimal risk of precipitating
a withdrawal reaction (ie, to at least 5 days after the last opiate use) but no
later than day 21 of the study. Subjects who passed the naloxone challenge
and started naltrexone on days 11–21 were considered successful detoxifications. Those who returned to using opiates and failed to begin naltrexone by
day 21 were considered unsuccessful.

Successful detoxification and induction onto naltrexone was accomplished with ten of the fifteen subjects. All patients rated lofexidine as
moderately to extremely effective in reducing most of the commonly
experienced withdrawal symptoms: insomnia, lethargy, and muscle/bone pain
were the most frequent residual complaints. None of the ten subjects reported
unacceptable withdrawal symptoms while taking lofexidine. Those who failed
to complete the detoxification procedure cited opiate craving rather than
withdrawal discomfort as the major reason for returning to opiate use. None
of the subjects reported ovesedation, dizziness, or lightheadedness from
lofexidine, despite rapid increases in the dose to as much as 1.6 mg per day
within the first 5 days. The maximum daily lofexidine dose ranged from 0.6
mg to 1.6 mg across the ten subjects with an average of 1.2 mg. There was
no significant lowering of blood pressure even at the maximum lofexidine
dose (mean prelofexidine BP; 115/74 mmHg: mean BP at maximum
lofexidine dose; 115/76 mmHg). Dry mouth and mild drowsiness were the
most commonly reported side effects. Reductions in the daily lofexidine
dose by 0.2 to 0.6 mg per day at the end of the study produced no symptomatic complaints or significant changes in blood pressure.

DISCUSSION

While our studies of clonidine suggest the usefulness of this non-opiate agent in outpatient opiate detoxification, it has also become clear that clonidine is not without clinical risks and potential drawbacks and thus is not an ideal agent for treating withdrawal symptoms. Some patients are extremely sensitive to clonidine's hypotensive and sedative effects and cannot tolerate the doses needed to relieve withdrawal discomfort. This has led patients to discontinue their detoxification before completion and has seriously restricted the usefulness of clonidine in outpatient withdrawal to patients whose level of opiate dependence is below 30 mg/day of methadone. Additionally, the close monitoring of patients that is required because of potentially troublesome side effects during clonidine treatment can be inordinately time-consuming and inconvenient for both patient and physician. These factors tend to decrease the efficacy and acceptability of clonidine detoxification especially in an outpatient setting where side effects can interfere with the patient's daily functioning.

Our results with lofexidine suggest that this medication is comparable to clonidine in terms of antiwithdrawal efficacy but without the adverse sedative and hypotensive side effects that limit clonidine's usefulness. It appears, therefore, that lofexidine might be a more clinically useful and viable treatment than clonidine in opiate detoxification, especially with ambulatory outpatients where safety and ability to maintain normal functioning are important concerns. Additionally, because lofexidine can be administered in higher doses than clonidine without unacceptable side effects, it might be possible to detoxify outpatients from higher levels of opiate dependence than has been the case with clonidine.

Non-opiate treatment with clonidine or lofexidine may be specifically indicated and preferable to detoxification using methadone in some cases. For example, these agents may be the treatment of choice for addicts with low levels of opiate dependence whose addiction might be increased by the use of methadone.

Clonidine or lofexidine may be especially useful in treating iatrogenic addiction to prescription opiates and treating addicted physicians or others having no prior involvement with illicit opiates where exposure to methadone or methadone treatment facilities might be undesirable or contraindicated. In general, clonidine and lofexidine may provide potentially useful and desirable treatment options whenever detoxification using methadone is inappropriate, unsuccessful, or simply unavailable.

Clonidine and lofexidine seem best suited for clinical use as transitional treatments between opiate dependence and naltrexone. Non-opiate medications with significant withdrawal-suppressing effects can provide symptomatic relief following rapid discontinuation of opiates without postponing the introduction of naltrexone at the earliest possible time to foster continued abstinence. The treatment sequence of clonidine or lofexidine followed as soon as possible by naltrexone induction is highly attractive to outpatients because it offers the opportunity for rapid detoxification with minimal discomfort and a clearly defined endpoint to the detoxification process.

The role of detoxification treatment alone as a therapeutic modality has long been overemphasized in addiction treatment. Attempts to detoxify large numbers of opiate addicts using clonidine or lofexidine and based on expectations that these patients will remain abstinent without some form of intensive aftercare treatment are highly unrealistic. In most cases, readdiction will rapidly ensue. Addicts are extremely vulnerable to relapse, particularly during the first week or two following cessation of opiate use. Although clonidine and lofexidine might be extremely useful in helping addicts achieve initial abstinence, a more comprehensive multimodality aftercare treatment approach including naltrexone and psychotherapy is usually necessary in enabling detoxified addicts to maintain an abstinent state (Resnick et al, 1981).

ACKNOWLEDGMENTS

The authors' research studies cited in this paper were conducted in a treatment program at New York Medical College sponsored by the New York State Office of Alcoholism and Substance Abuse, Division of Substance Abuse Services. Research funds were provided by the National Institute on Drug Abuse and Merrell-Dow Pharmaceuticals, Inc.

REFERENCES

Gold MS, Redmond DE and Kleber HD: Clonidine blocks acute opiate-withdrawal symptoms. *Lancet* 1:599–601, 1978

Maner T, Mehra J, Johnson C et al: Comparative efficacy of two centrally acting imidazoline derivatives, clonidine and lofexidine. *Clin Res* 28:33A, 1980

Rawson RA, Washton AM, Resnick RB et al: Clonidine hydrochloride detoxification from methadone treatment: The value of naltrexone aftercare. In: Harris LS (ed) *Problems of Drug Dependence, 1980.* DHHS, Publication No. (ADM) 81-1058. NIDA Research Monograph No. 34, pp 101–108, 1981

Resnick RB, Schuyten-Resnick E and Washton AM: Narcotic antagonists in the treatment of opioid dependence: Review and commentary. *Comp Psychiatry* 20:116–125, 1979

Resnick RB, Washton AM, Stone-Washton N et al: Psychotherapy and naltrexone in opioid dependence. In: Harris LS (ed) *Problems of Drug Dependence, 1980.*

Department of Health and Human Services, Publication No. (ADM) 81-1058. NIDA Research Monograph No. 34. Washington: U.S. Government Printing Office, pp 109–115, 1981

Shearman GT, Lal H and Ursillo RC: Effectiveness of lofexidine in blocking morphine-withdrawal signs in the rat. *Pharmacol Biochem Behav* 12:573–575, 1980

St. John LaCorte W, Jain AK, Ryan JR et al: Comparative efficacy and tolerability of lofexidine and clonidine given alone or concomitantly with hydrochlorathiazide in hypertensive outpatients. *Clin Pharmacol Ther* 29:259, 1981

Washton AM and Resnick RB: Clonidine for opiate detoxification: Outpatient clinical trials. *Am J Psychiatry* 137:1121–1122, 1980a

Washton AM and Resnick RB: Clonidine in opiate withdrawal: Review and appraisal of clinical findings. *Pharmacotherapy* 1(2):140–146, 1981

Washton AM and Resnick RB: Clonidine versus methadone for opiate detoxification. *Lancet* 2:1297, 1980b

Washton AM, Resnick RB and LaPlaca R: Clonidine hydrochloride: A nonopiate treatment for opiate withdrawal. *Psychopharm Bull* 2:50–52, 1980a

Washton AM, Resnick RB, Perzel JF and Garwood J: Lofexidine, a clonidine analogue effective in opiate withdrawal. *Lancet* I:991–992, 1981

Washton AM, Resnick RB and Rawson RA: Clonidine for outpatient opiate detoxification. *Lancet* 1:1078–1079, 1980b

19

The Swedish Methadone Maintenance Program

LARS M. GUNNE
LEIF GRÖNBLADH

BACKGROUND AND CLINICAL CONSIDERATIONS

In Sweden the intravenous abuse of illegally obtained opiates has been a gradually increasing problem since the mid-sixties, but it has not yet reached American proportions. For a couple of decades amphetamine and other central stimulants were dominating the Swedish drug market. Among the opiates raw opium was the leading drug in the early seventies, to be replaced first by morphine base and since 1975 by heroin. In a recent case-finding survey (Olsson, 1981) it has been estimated that Sweden has 3,000 to 4,000 users of heroin, about half of whom are regular users with a compulsive type of dependence on this drug.

The Swedish methadone maintenance treatment (MMT) system, which was set up at our clinic in 1966, has so far remained the only national MMT program and has received applicants from the whole country. Due to the differences in dimensions and intensity between the United States and Sweden, we have felt that we might proceed and develop our treatment program at a slow pace and with a greater amount of caution than was possible when American mega-programs were being organized.

Our aim has been to reserve the Swedish MMT program for a certain category of heroin abusers, as defined by a drug career model (Frykholm and Gunne, 1980). We have found that drug abusers tend to make use of treatment facilities in a manner that changes gradually as they move from one stage to another in their drug career. In the early stages they characteristically enter clinics for reasons other than to become permanently drug free. These patients tend to stay in treatment only for a few days, mainly in order to

205

receive substitution medication. When this medication is reduced to a point where they no longer feel comfortable, they typically leave against medical advice. This category of patients might be interested in long-lasting MMT, but we have tried to avoid them by insisting that they should try to live without drugs.

Later in the drug career the patients' treatment goals change and they may actually be striving to rid themselves of drugs on a permanent basis. At this stage their visits to the clinic may be prolonged past the acute withdrawal phase and the drug-free periods after discharge indicate an improved pattern. We try not to interfere at this stage either, but rather to leave the patient to his drug-free treatment programs, of which there are many nowadays in Sweden. Unfortunately, there is no reliable information regarding the success rate in those treatment systems, but at least some heroin addicts apparently manage to abandon their drug habit at this stage, with or without treatment.

Only when a heroin addict has a history of long-term compulsive abuse with repeated failures to stop, in spite of documented serious attempts to do so, then he becomes eligible for the Swedish MMT program. In order to select drug abusers according to the goals and aims described we have found the original eligibility criteria used by Dole and Nyswander (1965) to be quite useful and have maintained them unaltered over the 15 years our program has been in operation. These criteria are: (1) a history of at least four years of compulsive regular i.v. use of heroin, as documented by earlier hospital records; (2) at least three completed detoxifications, the patient must have remained in the clinic for more than a week after all drugs have been discontinued; (3) withdrawal signs and urinary opioid excretion on admission; (4) at least 20 years of age; (5) not arrested, not serving sentence; (6) no dominating abuse of non-opiate drugs.

EVALUATION RESEARCH

The evaluation of an MMT system ideally should contain these four elements:

(1) A comparison of the subjects' situation *before* vs *during* (or after) treatment

(2) Comparison between yearly results, to check for the *stability* of the program

(3) Comparison between treated and untreated (or alternatively treated) assigned by random allocation to control for effects of *selection* and *self-selection*

(4) Long-term effects of methadone (which is not covered in the present paper).

In an ongoing evaluation study (Grönbladh, 1982) the effects of our MMT program on work, criminality rate and drug abuse is carried out. Table 1 shows the number of weeks our patients have worked two years and one year before they were accepted in the MMT program, together with the corresponding figures for the first and second year in treatment. The total material of 170 cases (131 male, 39 female) was subdivided into those who are still in treatment, those who have been voluntarily discharged, involuntarily discharged, and those who have died while in treatment. The number of weeks of employed increased from 2-8 before treatment to around 33 weeks during the second year of treatment, except in the group which was later discharged involuntarily, due to continued abuse of amphetamines and/or hypnotics.

A measurement of the stability of the program is exemplified in Figure 1. When work rehabilitation was measured for seven consecutive years it was found that the percentage of individuals who were working or studying varied between 59-81 percent. In addition, a percentage of able-bodied subjects were reporting to the employment exchange agency as willing to accept any job that might be offered. The sum of these three categories varied between 83 and 91 percent, who were thus able and willing to work. The program stability with regard to work rehabilitation was considered to be satisfactory.

EFFECTS OF SELECTION

It has been argued in the Swedish debate about our results that the subjects selected for treatment by our criteria might represent a group which could be on their way out of the drug career anyway and thus perhaps not in need of MMT, which might even prolong their period of dependence on opiates. In order to elucidate this question we carried out a comparative study of two groups, which were both eligible according to our criteria but

Table 1. Weeks of Employment/Year (Means ± S.E.) Among 170 Subjects in the Swedish MMT Program

	N	2 Years Before	1 Year Before	First Year	Second Year
In program	96	1.9 ± 0.6	3.3 ± 0.9	27 ± 2	33 ± 2 (n = 67)
Voluntary discharge	28	5.7 ± 3	6.0 ± 2	20 ± 4	32 ± 5 (n = 20)
Compulsory discharge	37	1.9 ± 0.9	4.1 ± 1	6.1 ± 2	8.9 ± 2 (n = 19)
Deceased	9	5.9 ± 2	7.7 ± 3	18 ± 8	34 ± 9 (n = 7)

Per cent

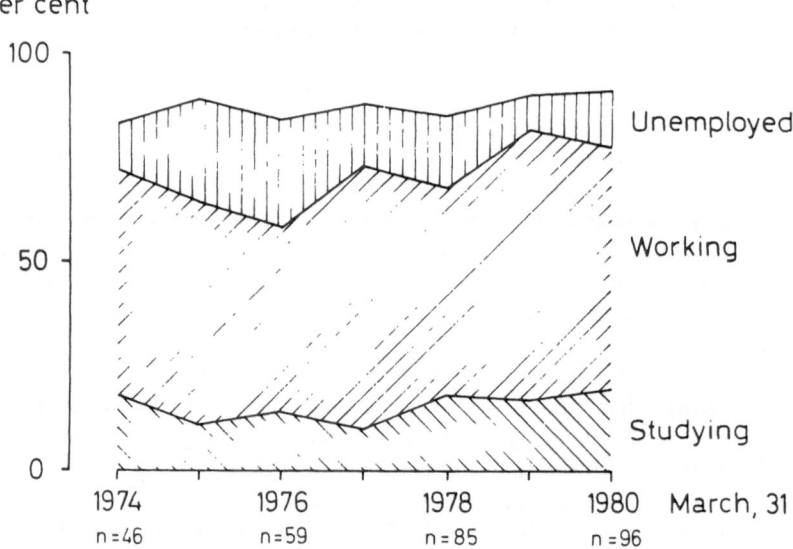

Fig. 1. Yearly percentage of studying, working, and unemployed (reporting employment exchange agencies) during the years 1974–1980. Numbers of individuals (n) given in the figure

where one, by random assignment, did not receive MMT. All subjects participating in this study were between ages 20 and 24 and physically healthy when they applied for MMT. The study was carried on until the difference between pairs was significant on a five percent level using sequential analysis according to Bross (1952), which occurred after 34 individuals has been included. Details of the methodology have been given elsewhere (Gunne and Grönbladh, 1981).

Figure 2 illustrates the situation before the start of the experiment. Each circle represents an individual (H in the circle stands for regular heroin abuse). To the left are the 17 who will be given methadone, to the right there are 17 who, by random allocation, will not be given this treatment. Table 2 shows that the mean age, number of years of drug abuse, number of treatment periods, and court trials was about the same in both groups. Only the sex distribution differed, the experimental group having six females as compared to two in the control group.

A refusal to accept a patient in our MMT program means that the subject cannot apply again until two years later. For that reason the situation after two years is of interest (before any of the controls had an

Before

| Experimental group (methadone) | Control group (no methadone) |

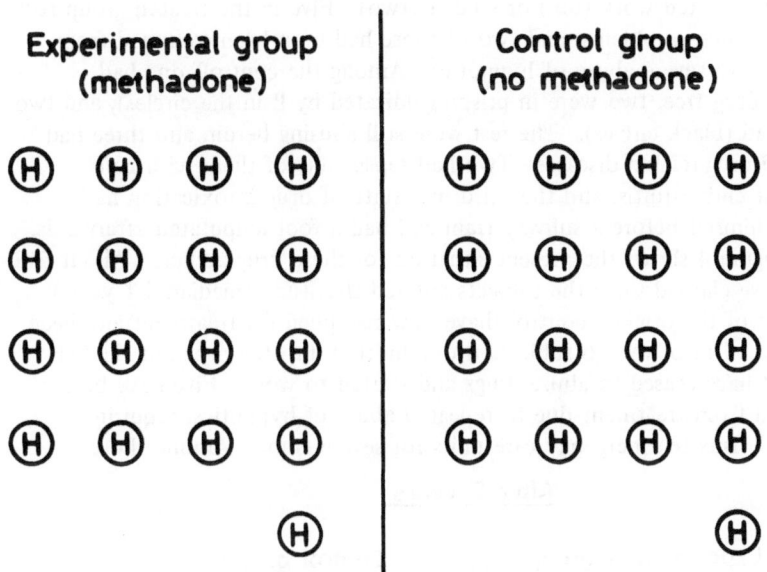

Fig. 2. Situation before the randomization study: each circle represents an individual 20–24 yrs old. H in the circles stands for regular I.V. heroin abuse. Left half: experimental group which will be accepted for MMT; Right half: controls, which will not be given MMT

Table 2. Some Background Data Within the Experimental
and Control Groups Before Admission

	Experimental (n = 17)	Control (n = 17)	
Sex	11 m. 6 f.	15 m. 2 f.	
Age	22.9 ± 1.3 yrs	22.5 ± 1.2 yrs	Mean ± SD
Drug abuse, duration	7.5 ± 1.8 yrs	7.5 ± 1.9 yrs	Mean ± SD
I.V. heroin, duration	6.6 ± 1.5 yrs	6.6 ± 1.2 yrs	
Inpatient treatment*	13.8 (4–25) periods	14.4 (4–20) periods	Median (range)
Court trials	4.5 (0–8) times	4.8 (0–8) times	Median (range)
Work during last year	2 Sporadically	None	

*Including mental hospitals, treatment homes, self-regulating communities, foster homes
and family care, but excluding intensive care units, internal medicine clinics, etc.

opportunity to enter the treatment program). Figure 3 shows that after two years 12 of the patients given methadone had abandoned their drug abuse and started work (ten) or studies (two). Five in the treated group still had drug abuse problems, and two of those had even been excluded from MMT due to severe abuse of hypnotics. Among the controls one had become drug free, two were in prison (indicated by P in the circles), and two were dead (black circles). The rest were still abusing heroin and three had incurred drug-related diseases. Two had sepsis, one of them with concomitant endocarditis, and the third in a state of drug intoxication had thrown himself before a subway train and had a foot amputated afterwards.

Figure 4 shows the present situation for these drug addicts. About five years have elapsed since the subjects entered the study (median 5.1 years) and nine of the original controls have now reapplied for treatment and been accepted. Out of the 26 subjects thus admitted into the program, 21 (81 percent) have ceased to abuse drugs and started to work. Five have been excluded from treatment due to repeated abuse of hypnotics, requiring repeated visits to emergency care units for severe coma. Among those

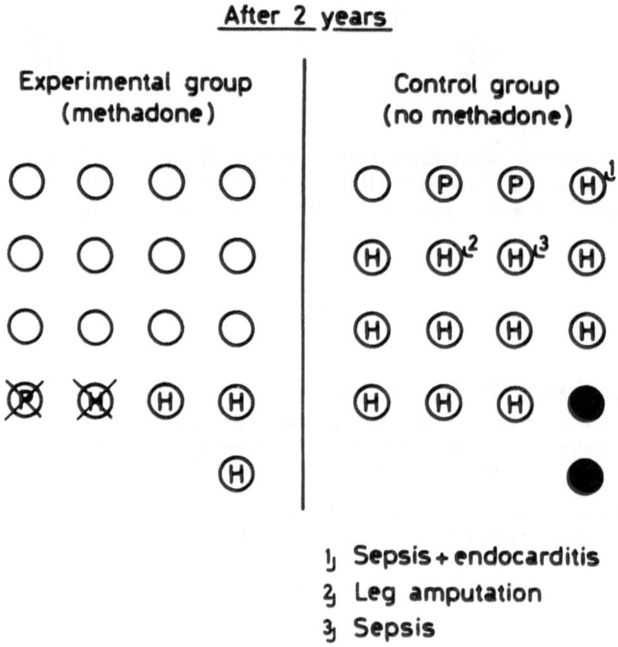

After 2 years

Experimental group
(methadone)

Control group
(no methadone)

1) Sepsis + endocarditis
2) Leg amputation
3) Sepsis

Fig. 3. Situation 2 yrs after acceptance or decline. White circle: no drug abuse. H in circle: abuse of heroin or (in the experimental group) hypnotics. P in circle: subject in prison. Black circle: deceased. Crossed circle means that the patient has been expelled from treatment

Present situation

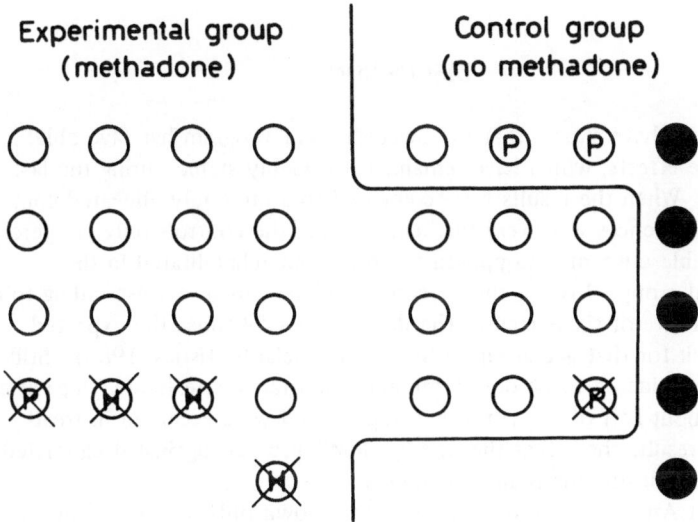

Fig. 4. Present situation: nine within the original control group have been accepted in the MMT program. For an explanation of symbols, see Fig. 3

subjects who have not received MMT, five are dead (allegedly from overdose), two in prison and one is still drug free.

Table 3 compares the results within the original experimental group of 17 with the outcome of the entire MMT program of 170. It is seen that the percentage of successful cases (free of drug abuse and in treatment plus drug free after voluntary discharge from the program) is quite similar between

Table 3. Distribution of the Experimental Group
in Three Different Categories at the End of Experiment,
and the Size of the Corresponding Categories Within the Total MMT Program

	Experimental (n = 17)	Total Program (n = 170)
In program (no drug abuse)	64%	58%
Voluntarily left MMT (drug free)	12%	14%
Involuntarily detoxification (current abuse)	24%	20%*
Other categories	–	8%

*The death rate within this category is under investigation.

the two groups. Thus, from the point of view of outcome, the experimental group proved to be a representative sample of the total program.

DISCUSSION

Our data have shown that the Swedish MMT program has favorable rehabilitative effects, which have remained reasonably stable during the last seven years. When the results were compared to a randomly allocated control group the differences were very marked. Among the controls only six percent had a favorable outcome as opposed to 76 percent rehabilitated in the experimental group. Five of the 17 control subjects died, corresponding to a yearly death rate of six percent. The death rate is 59 times the expected mortality risk for that age group in Sweden (Official Statistics, 1980). Still it must be considered to be only a minimum mortality rate figure, since after two years about half of the controls reapplied and were accepted in treatment. The results show that the Swedish MMT protects against drug-related morbidity and death among heroin addicts.

Recent American outcome research has shown only a marginal or no effect when MMT is compared with drug-free treatment or no treatment (Sells and Simpson, 1979; Burt et al, 1980). This difference between the Swedish and some American treatment operations, probably has to do with the selection of cases. Due to our restrictive admission policy the Swedish program is being regarded as a last resort among heroin addicts. Those who are accepted are thus likely to put a maximal effort in their own rehabilitation, a tendency that is further amplified by the therapists' emphasis on patients' employment and work. All this may contribute to the favorable outcome, which seems to be comparable to the pioneering American MMT programs (Dole et al, 1968).

ACKNOWLEDGMENTS

This study has been supported by a Medical Research Council grant nr 4810. The design of the randomization study was approved by the Swedish Board of Health and Welfare and by the Ethics' Committee of the University of Uppsala.

REFERENCES

Bross I: Sequential medical plans. *Biometrics* 1988–205, 1952

Burt MR, Brown BS and DuPont RL: Follow-up of former clients of a large multi-modality drug treatment program. *Int J Addict* 15:391–408, 1980

Dole VP and Nyswander M: A medical treatment for diacetylmorphine (heroin) addiction. *JAMA* 193:646–650, 1965

Dole VP, Nyswander M and Warner A: Successful treatment of 750 criminal addicts. *JAMA* 206:2708–11, 1968

Frykholm B and Gunne L-M: Studies of the drug career. *Acta Psychiat Scand* 62 (suppl 284):42–51, 1980

Gunne L-M and Grönbladh L: The Swedish methadone maintenance program: A controlled study. *Drug Alc Dep* 1981

Olsson B: National case-finding study in Sweden ICAA report. (In press) 1981

Sells B and Simpson D: Bulletin on Narcotics, Vol. XXXI No. 1, 1979

20

The Odyssey House Treatment Method

JUDIANNE DENSEN-GERBER

GENERAL STATEMENT

Odyssey House, Inc, is a voluntary nonprofit agency which began as a pilot research program at Metropolitan Hospital in January, 1966. At that time, Dr. A. Ronald Sorvino was assigned the task of evaluating the use of the maintenance drug, cyclazocine. Based on his prior unsuccessful experience with methadone drug maintenance alone, Dr. Sorvino asked me as resident psychiatrist assigned to the ward, to develop a long-term psychotherapeutic setting in which the narcotic addict might be more responsive to psychiatric intervention.

Subsequently, in early January 1966 I visited with Dr. Efren Ramirez in Rio Piedras, Puerto Rico. Impressed with his work, I agreed to try to adapt his method to the New York City milieu. Odyssey House is the successful outgrowth of that project. We now serve fourteen American states, two in Australia, and the countries of New Zealand and Israel in the field of drug and substance abuse.

Historically, in August 1966 the patients influenced the doctors in charge of the program to conclude that continuance of the maintenance concept gave the antitherapeutic message that the patients were crippled and unable to function normally without drugs. The patients requested discontinuance of cyclazocine. However, a drug-free project, no matter the promise it showed, was incompatible with Metropolitan Hospital's commitment to drug testing. Therefore, the patients were discharged from the hospital in October 1966.

Seventeen of them elected to continue the work of the therapeutic community. Their dedication to the belief that they could function without drugs, that they could be successfully treated by psychiatric intervention, and that they had a responsibility to prevent, through education and example, the spreading and continuation of addiction, rallied many members of the community to aid and assist them. Three psychiatrists volunteered their services free of charge in the initial interim period. At the same time, a small seven-room building was loaned to them. Until June 1967 the group was self-sustaining, supported minimally by donations.

In March 1967 Odyssey House was incorporated and soon received tax-exemption from the Internal Revenue Service. Its strong belief in the therapeutic community method of treating addictive diseases, based on the statistics of the Rio Piedras experience and its own high success rate, committed Odyssey House to the expansion of its program to meet the compelling needs of the community. A voluntary agency has the important ability of being sufficiently flexible to develop, test, and modify its ideas and methods. The small professional staff is dedicated to the observation, recording, and analyzing of the treatment data accumulated. Every session in the community is recorded for future research evaluation.

In order to expand, in May 1967 Odyssey House rented a building at 309-311 East 6 Street in Manhattan. These quarters have facilities for approximately sixty persons—forty males and twenty females—plus eight resident ex-addict staff. Odyssey House occupied these premises in early June 1967.

Within the next year Odyssey House grew quickly, responding to the desire of more and more drug addicts to enter treatment. A motivational facility was opened in Harlem and a "re-entry house" in the Bronx was leased to Odyssey by the Roman Catholic Church for $1 per year.

By March 1969 Odyssey House had facilities for 130 residents and was continuously overcrowded. One of the causes for the overcrowding was the great number of teenagers seeking admission to the program. It was at this time that the Odyssey staff spearheaded the public outcry against the rising number of teenagers becoming addicted to heroin in New York City. The Deputy Chief Medical Examiner of the City of New York grimly confirmed this trend as he reported almost one teenage death daily in New York City from heroin.

Reluctantly, governmental officials decided to recognize the problem, but not before Odyssey House took the initiative and opened an adolescent treatment unit totally dependent on private funds. Technically, this was illegal, since Odyssey House did not possess an appropriate Certificate of Occupancy and the Odyssey House Charter did not allow for treatment of patients under 16.

In 1971 the Odyssey Method was adapted to treat addicted parents in addition to adults and adolescents. The outgrowth of this project is the Parents Program—the only treatment facility in the United States where children up to the age of five can be in residence with their parents: the children have round-the-clock supervision, medical care, and a diversified school/play program; the parents take part in a traditional Odyssey treatment program, but which emphasizes learning child nurturing skills. The major goal of the Parents Program is to break the multigenerational cycle of drug abuse and child abuse/neglect.

The Odyssey method of treatment is unique in that it is an easily understandable and teachable process of changing a person's behavior and basic attitudes. The flexibility of the Odyssey Method is demonstrated in its successful application in such diverse social milieu as Louisiana, Maine, Michigan, New Hampshire, and Utah, as well as in Australia, New Zealand, and Israel.

In spite of rather phenomenal growth, Odyssey House has been able to maintain high standards of excellence in therapy because of close supervision by an independent team of specialists four times a year, both for program control and modification.

The rehabilitation service program is divided into three phases: (1) pre-treatment or induction, (2) intensive residential treatment and (3) post-treatment or re-entry. Induction is divided into three stages; first, awareness of the program's existence; second, the motivation of the street addict to enter treatment accomplished while he remains in the community; and third, the first in-residence challenge, the candidacy-in, to determine the sincerity of his motivation.

The treatment phase is divided into three levels discussed more fully (see also Program Flow Chart, pp 218–219). The post-treatment phase is also divided into three stages: the in-residence one of level IV, during which time the patient begins resocialization; candidacy-out, accomplished in the community with the patient's return for after-care only; and finally, discharge to out-patient status. This concept is known as *the rule of three upon three.*

INDUCTION: PRE-TREATMENT PHASE

The initial presenting problem after the addict learns about the program's existence is that the raw street addict has a tenacious hold on street values called the code of the street. It represents to him the only code for survival remaining to follow. This hold not only supports him in his rebellion against organized society, but also strangles any effort of his to seek and benefit from conventional treatment. He is unable to interact in a patient-

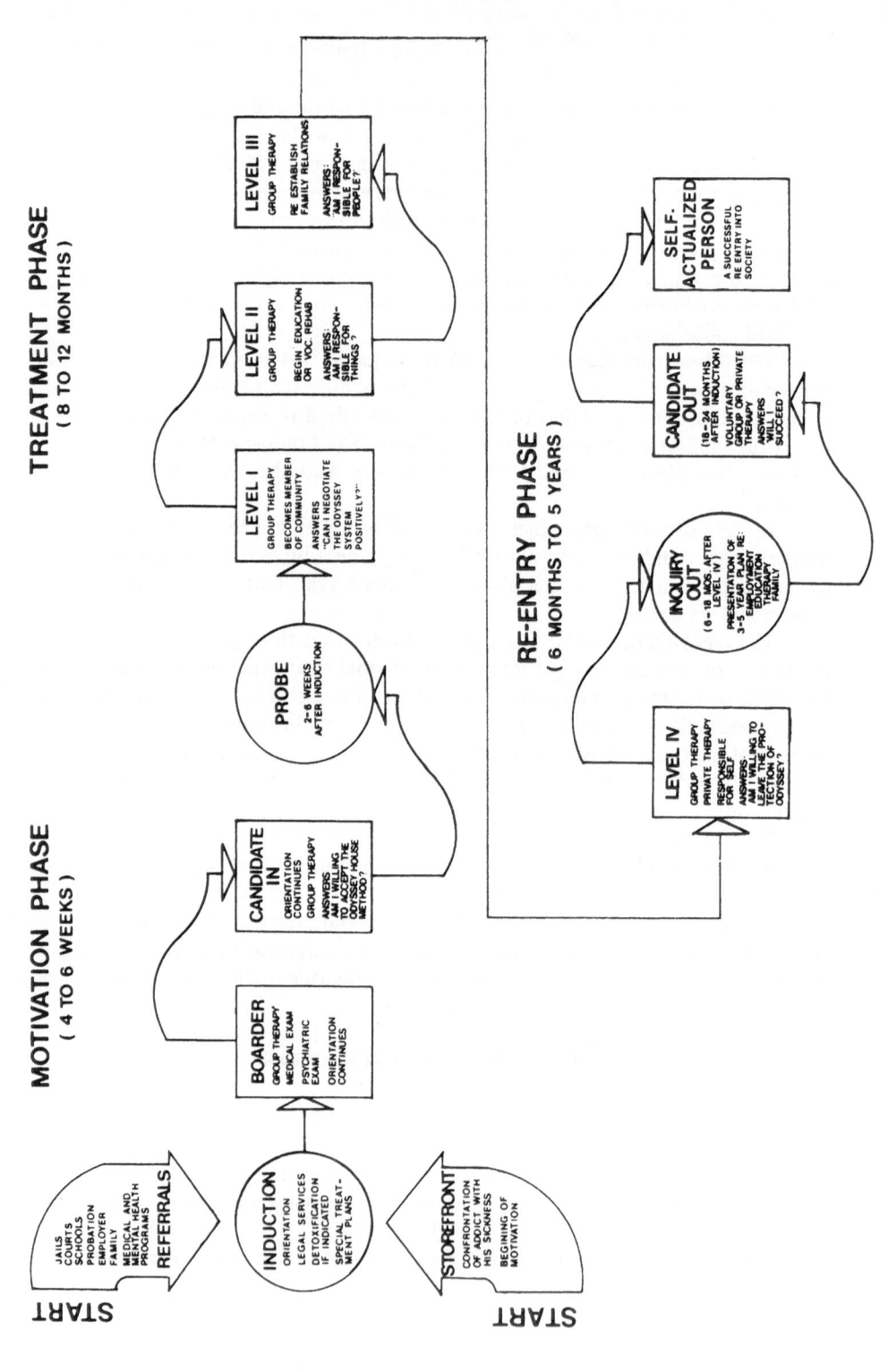

BOARDER

The resident is now living within the treatment facility. During the next 48 hour period, he or she receives a complete medical examination and a psychiatric evaluation (a full battery of psychological tests will be given within 45 to 60 days after admission). A treatment plan is designed for the patient and appended to his/her chart. Detoxification is begun for pregnant addicts, methadone addicts and barbiturate addicts only.

CANDIDATE-IN

Candidate-In is a 4-6 week period in which the resident learns to discipline him or herself and become more familiar with the treatment process. Candidates In are responsible for manual labor and behaving themselves. They have no status and are working towards acceptance into the community.

Peer acceptance is a prime force in treating the drug abuser. Once deviant behavior is no longer rewarded by the peer group, the new resident then faces either exclusion by the group or must orient him or herself toward positive behavior.

The resident must decide "Do I want Odyssey?"

PROBE

The probe is an intensive group session in which the new resident is probed by representative members of each level of the program and a professional staff member. The resident must recognize and admit that he or she is sick, is in need of treatment and accepts the Odyssey method and the doctor-patient relationship. If the resident can answer in the affirmative, (s)he is moved to Level I. If not, the resident must begin the motivational stage again from the beginning.

LEVEL I

The resident for the first time is an accepted member with a voice in the community. Emphasis is now placed on attitudes and the formation of positive interpersonal relationships. All activities, whether they be work or play, are done in group settings. The Level I begins to verbalize feelings and to trust in the group process. When the resident has proven to be capable of negotiating the Odyssey House system positively, (s)he moves to Level II.

LEVEL II

For the first time, the resident is an authority figure. Since drug abusers have great contempt for authority, they do not begin to deal with this problem until they are placed in a responsible position of authority. Emphasis is placed on the organization and administration of tasks. They learn by doing and they learn to evaluate what they do.

LEVEL III

The Level III residents are given the responsibility for the well-being of those under their authority. They are learning to be responsible for people and to become a strength within the community by guiding residents through the rehabilitation process. They set the example of appropriate attitudes and behavior for residents in the motivation and treatment phases. They become co-therapists and act as a bridge between the professional therapist and the new resident.

The Level III begins to re-establish relationships with his/her family on occassional weekend passes, and for the first time, is allowed to leave the facility unescorted.

When the Level III has proven to be responsible for people (s)he is moved to Level IV.

LEVEL IV

As a Level IV, the resident assumes a quasi-staff position within the community. He or she receives a small stipend and evenings off with a curfew. Group therapy is continued and the Level IV may enter private therapy if necessary. The first six months of Level IV are spent living and working in the Odyssey community. The Level IV is giving back to the community what he or she received from Odyssey.

At the end of this period, the Level IV must live apart from the Odyssey community and may begin to attend college, vocational training programs or obtain a job outside of Odyssey.

If the Level IV is observed by staff to be coping positively in a mature manner, he/she is proposed for Candidate-Out.

INQUIRY-OUT

The proposed Level IV must have a high school diploma, a driver's license and a promise of employment in order to graduate. He or she must present a realistic 3-5 year plan covering future employment, education, follow-up therapy (if necessary), and living arrangements. If this plan is satisfactory to his/her peers, Odyssey graduates and staff, he or she then becomes a Candidate-Out.

CANDIDATE-OUT

The graduate is now independent of the Odyssey community and is engaging in a healthy life style in the community at large. Friendships are developed. The career is extended and the individual learns to answer. "Can I succeed?" affirmatively. Follow-up groups are conducted bi-monthly in the evening as a problem solving source for any difficulties encountered.

SELF-ACTUALIZED PERSON

The self-actualized person is a fully functioning, constructive member of society and can "face the future unafraid." The individual is free of all major psycopathology and can problem solve without fear of returning to a self-destructive life style.

doctor relationship, even if his initial indifference, skepticism, and negativism can be overcome.

The pre-treatment phase is designed to motivate the street addict to enter into a meaningful therapeutic endeavor. Its primary function is to pave the way for the future doctor-patient relationship. The extreme importance of this is obvious to any professional who has been the object of the reactive contempt the addict initially shows towards the non-addict world, because of his own psychopathology of isolation, loneliness, and low self-esteem. However, within most addicts is the faint, but real, desire to return to functioning in a positive manner. Therefore, the first constructive therapeutic relationship is, by necessity, that of an ex-addict group leader to a raw street addict.

The street addict, called by Odyssey the raw addict, may enter treatment on his own initiative or be sent from another referring agency, either private or public. The Induction Supervisor screens and accepts for admission addicts who are in prison, on the request of their counsel, by court order, or through the parole division of the Department of Correction. He has secured special permission to enter the facilities of the Department of Correction. The source of referral is unimportant, as long as the raw addict is exposed to the first motivational phase. However, the Induction Supervisor reserves the right to refuse admission to any applicant. The overwhelming majority of drug addicts are not psychotic. They are legally and psychiatrically responsible for the consequences of their actions and should be held accountable. Experience has shown that those addicts who are incarcerated by the law, or who feel incarcerated, or who are unwilling to accept treatment voluntarily, will be amenable to treatment when a proper pre-treatment phase is instituted.

The youthful addict or drug abuser under the age of 18 is accepted immediately into the program at any time, regardless of whether he has used drugs within the past few hours. The older addict must show sufficient (although quite minimal) motivation before he will be allowed to enter treatment. This is achieved by displaying a cooperative attitude, appearing on time for induction, and decreasing his addiction to a point where he can enter the residence without requiring detoxification. No addictive substances are permitted or prescribed within the residences.

For most patients detoxification has not been found to be necessary. Severe withdrawal is a rarity; all residents spend their first seventy-two hours in the program with a "buddy" and are closely watched by physicians and registered nurses as well as trained ex-addict supervisors.

When the raw addict is considered by the ex-addict team ready for admission to the community for the second stage of induction, the candidacy-in, he is sponsored by the level IV co-leader to the ex-addict and medical treatment supervisors of the intensive treatment unit. Either one can refuse admission, returning the applicant to the beginning groups for further motivational work.

In addition, the previously described method of admission is therapeutic for the level IV residents. It exposes them to the confrontation of the street values, beyond which they have now grown. This confrontation or challenge occurs at the beginning of their own resocialization and re-entry into the general community, the initial weaning from the protective isolation of the residence. The Induction Supervisor is continuing not only his confrontation with the addicts in the street, but also, he is assuming the responsibility of training others, the level IV residents, to undertake responsibility. He is increasing his sphere of authority. His staff is responsible for summarizing all the contacts with the patients during this first stage and beginning the resident's individual chart.

Within twenty-four hours of admission to Odyssey House, the second phase of induction is begun, "The Candidacy-In." This is initiated by an Inquiry-In, which is conducted by the House Coordinator in conjunction with representatives from the entire community. The functions of this meeting are to familiarize and acquaint the resident-patients with the proposed new member, to take a complete history, and to afford him a constructive sense of belonging. An additional purpose is to identify, as quickly as possible, any major problem areas which later may complicate the interpersonal in-residence relationships.

The Inquiry-In is for the benefit of both the patient himself and the community, not only to enable the group to function better therapeutically, but also to be protected from and to cope with the inevitable gaming and testing behavior which has a unique flavor with each resident. The Inquiry-In openly confronts the patient with the expectations and demands of the community upon him as regards his behavior, and the consequences which will ensue from negative behavior. That such consequences must ensue without the possibility of mitigation is essential to the growth of these patients.

The breaking of any of four cardinal rules means immediate expulsion from the residence. These are: the use of contraband; stealing; a threat or act of physical violence; and any sexual acting out, whether heterosexual or homosexual in nature. The latter three rules are enforced by the senior patients and staff. The first is not left to the clinical evaluation of the other patients and staff.

In order to ascertain with certainty that the residents and staff are drug-free, their urines are analyzed on a daily basis and certified to be free of all substances such as opiates, barbiturates, hypnotics, and amphetamines, by an independent laboratory.

The Inquiry-In constitutes the first formal community challenge to the addict. It tests sincerity and motivational drive. It is a clear demonstration of the positive constructive functioning of the therapeutic community. The patient is shown dramatically that the community means business. A copy of the Inquiry-In, plus comments from the resident-patients present, are appended to the chart. The patient is now a candidate-in.

The candidate-in is responsible for the major manual work within the community. He is supervised by a level III resident. The candidate-in has four and one-half hours a week of group work with a therapist and a senior level III in his facility.

The residential day is structured from waking in the morning until bedtime. Little opportunity for leisure time is afforded. Between three and six hours a day is allotted to group meetings. The candidate-in has no voting rights or voice in the running of the community.

The candidate-in is given a complete medical work-up within twenty-four hours, including not only a routine history and physical but also complete blood and serological testing, urinalysis, chest X-ray, TB skin testing, and EKG. All female residents are given a PAP test. There is a licensed physician and a registered nurse assigned to each facility. All medical problems are worked up under the direction of the full-time Medical Director. The Medical Director also sees that each resident receives a complete psychiatric evaluation by a qualified psychiatrist within seventy-two hours of admission. Psychological testing is part of the general psychiatric evaluation. A complete medical and psychiatric report is appended to each resident's chart.

The Probe constitutes the next formal challenge to the candidate-in. When suitable progress has been made by the candidate-in, he may be sponsored by the treatment staff to become a full participating resident. The sponsorship must have the endorsement of the group leaders in charge of the proposed patient. The probe usually occurs within three to six weeks after the Inquiry-In. A candidate-in is entitled to one probe a week after his initial week within the community, or a single probe by default at the end of six weeks if he has not been sponsored. The probe is conducted by a member of the treatment staff and is attended by selected representatives from each higher in-residence level as well.

The function of the probe is for the candidate-in to prove to residents as well as the professional staff, by both word and deed, that he has a usable understanding of the concept of the house, and a commitment to live by it while in residential therapy. In reality, this means that the patient accepts the doctor-patient relationship that he is willing to look into himself for the answers to his problems, that he will accept responsibility for himself and his actions, and finally, that he will submit to authority and discipline of the community.

If he passes the probe, the candidate-in moves to level I. If there is one negative vote, in a sponsored probe, he remains a candidate-in; if the probe is by default, he is returned to the street addict groups for additional motivational work and future application for readmission to the House.

It is important that the program have value to the patients participating and to those considering admission. It must be preserved as an entity above and beyond any individual member. Therefore, there are times when a resident must be excluded from the community. It has been repeatedly demonstrated that confrontation and actualization of discharge have rededicated the majority of the persons affected, causing subsequent improved functioning on readmission.

If the candidate-in passes the probe, he is accepted as a full participating member. He now begins the intensive treatment phase per se. A copy of the probe, including comments by all those participating, is appended to the patient's chart.

TREATMENT PHASE

Now the addict begins in earnest the process of personality reorientation, or reconstruction. He comes relatively quickly to the realization that he is not a chronically sick person in need of drug maintenance, but rather that his way of life, or orientation towards functioning, is sick or distorted. It becomes very evident to him that his behavior is a result of free choice. No matter how deviant the past behavior of an addict has been, he has the innate capacity to function positively when properly challenged. The energies which before were destructive in nature are directed constructively in accord with those of society.

Acceptance by peers constitutes the prime force available in beginning therapy to the professional and ex-addict co-leader treating a group of sociopaths. Once deviant behavior is no longer rewarded by his group but has become grounds for exclusion, the speed with which new members are oriented to and accept positive, affirmative attitudes towards treatment, and adopt the senior members' judgment as to the therapist's qualifications is amazing. The therapist is an expert participant-guide in therapy meetings, but the patient participants are considered primarily responsible for the success or failure of any single endeavor. It is their work that counts, only they who stand to benefit from treatment or to lose if they game.

From its inception, the Odyssey House program is designed to create receptive peer-group relations, thereby permitting residents to relate to each other and the staff without fear of reprisal. There is no contraband in the house, no threat or actualization of physical violence, and "no contracts of silence" or "defending each other" in group therapy. The residents have assumed sole responsibility for the enforcement of the rules that they have instituted. This permits the treatment staff to devote full time to therapy rather than enforcing police or security methods. Thus, they are maximally able to utilize their training with minimum waste of effort, talent, or money. This prevents much of the frustration and depression often seen in professionals who treat addicts.

The emphasis in therapy is no present behavior, interpersonal relationships, and attitudes. The use of the past to excuse current behavior or to avoid present responsibility is discouraged. The past, for many of these patients is one of extreme deprivation, cruelty, and loneliness, at best. Much cannot be analyzed into acceptance through understanding and interpretation. It is explored and evaluated when of clear relevance, such as in incest trauma or unresolved oedipal conflicts. Stressed is resignation to the unchangeable reality of the patient's early life, a "now what" posture, coupled with an examination of what resources are present in the patient which he can tap to cope effectively in the here and now. The patient is challenged to begin today!

Excuses for poor functioning are not tolerated. The therapist is forcefully judgmental in his attitudes. To consider the patient, rather than his way of life, as sick, serves to reinforce the pathological defense of dependency on the part of the addict and the need of the professional to mother him.

The original Odyssey House core group of 17 addicts had "golden arms" worth one million, two hundred thousand dollars ($1,200,000) in illegal cost to society. This supported their actual yearly use of four hundred thousand dollars ($400,000). It is obvious upon reflection that they had the capacity to find room and board, to make and keep appointments, and hoodwink the most well-meaning, attuned professionals.

The inevitable conning, gaming, and manipulation is combatted by permitting group work only, and refusing all demands. This insistence on group work exclusively subjects each resident to the constant scrutiny of, and open confrontation by, his peers. No single resident can play one staff member against the other or against the community or vice-versa. This forces openness in therapy and prevents informing and gossip gathering. The only demands met by the staff are those of guidance and therapy. The professional is no longer a symbol of authority, police, or pill givers. There is a constant refusal to "do for", such as find jobs, education, or homes, but only to help them find themselves and group identity.

Thus, many of the basic pathologic features in the addict, his loneliness isolation, dependency and low self-esteem, are overcome. To recapitulate, the two cardinal prohibitions for the professional are no individual work and no demand meeting. It cannot be too greatly emphasized how little help the ex-addicts require. They take pride and "grow behind" doing for themselves. Whatever is accomplished has much more meaning and value to the patient under these circumstances and affords him the necessary stimulus for the required maturational growth. The Odyssey House techniques, though effective, have been difficult for many professionals to accept. They necessitate a relinquishing to the senior patient population, authority and responsibility, as well as according them respect. For it is respect for themselves and others that they must develop. This can be accomplished only through supervised, structured practice. The goal is positive, full functioning, independent people. It is difficult for many professionals to survive in the therapeutic community environment, because acceptance and status are accorded by the patients to a professional on the basis of his functioning as a real, warm, capable person, and not, on title per se. No one, neither patient nor worker, can demand respect, but each must earn it.

The concept of earning position and emotional growth through positive social interaction is deeply engrained in all the work. The residents are continually evaluated and re-evaluated bi-weekly by each other and monthly by the staff. It is partially on the basis of these evaluations that a resident will move from one level to another. The day of evaluation and phasing, is one of the most significant of the week. This minute subdividing or hierarchy creates additional incentive for positive growth, in accordance with the socially acceptable norms. The desire of an individual resident to win the approval of his peers and favorable recognition from an authority figure is clearly demonstrable.

Due to the severity of the psychopathology of drug addiction with its attendant social disruption to the lives of the addicts, it is felt that an in-residence setting is a prerequisite for successful treatment and that psychiatric intervention be intensive. All activities in the House are considered to be part of the therapy which is directed to returning the addict to normal living patterns. The residents are responsible for all the maintenance, laundry, cooking, office work, etc, which living demands of the rest of society. Nothing is done for them that they can do themselves. This serves three purposes: one, it teaches them that they can do for themselves; two, it gives them future job training such as typing, switchboard operation, bookkeeping, printing, etc; and last, but not least, it greatly reduces the cost of running the program.

In the past few years, several new group therapy forms have been developed, as well as the expansion and alteration of already existing methods. The attitude has been to test anything that seemed to offer promise, to discard nothing without a trial, to alter as deemed necessary and to accept on an empirical basis, if positive change occurred. There is a tacit commitment to being open, inventive and willing to learn from professional, ex-addict and resident alike.

Meeting forms which have evolved are as follows: business and general administrative meetings; concepts, either visual or verbal; special visitors meetings; regular group therapy sessions with a psychiatrist and alternates without; supervision of ex-addict co-leaders; encounters general, special, or marathon; orientation sessions for candidates-in, inquiries and probes; and phasing and evaluation with "feedback," to list only a few. It is impossible within the confines of this paper to describe the above in detail, but a representative from Odyssey House, if requested, would be glad to discuss any aspect of the program.

POST-TREATMENT OR RE-ENTRY PHASE

Reentry is divided into three stages. The first is that of level IV, then candidacy-out, and the last is discharge to out-patient status.

The transition from the protection of the resident unit, with its 16 hours a day therapeutic structured environment, to functioning within the community at large, is accomplished in supportive stages. It is begun by a level IV resident being proposed by his peers to the candidates-out and staff for an Inquiry-Out. This usually occurs after the resident has lived within the house for a period of twelve months and he is deemed by his peers to have experienced sufficient behavioral change and growth to cope with the demands of the street.

By referring to the therapy challenges at the different levels, one can see a slow developmental process unfold with increasing responsibilities and privileges. The candidate-in does most of the physical work, and has only motivational therapy. He must affirmatively answer the question: "Do I accept myself as a person needing help?" In level I, the number of therapy hours is doubled, with voting rights and a voice in the community afforded. He must learn the therapeutic techniques to help himself. He accepts that change will occur. In level II, the shift from predominately physical labor to office work is made with the development of certain vocational skills. He learns self-discipline by successfully completing tasks assigned to him. Supervised family visits are permitted. In level III, authority and leadership towards other residents is undertaken. He is permitted to travel alone on house business and receive unopened mail; he has earned trust when within the confines of the house. He attends therapy not only as a participant, but at times begins to assume co-leadership. He can head a small department. He learns to accept authority by being an authority figure. He is responsible for people.

Level IV begins with exodus out. He spends increasingly more time out of the house, meeting with the public, both formally at speaking engagements and informally whenever representing the house. He accompanies the Induction Supervisor in confronting and motivating the raw street addict in prisons, storefronts, or hospital settings. He assists the Treatment Supervisors in the running of the house by supervising general departments, and by co-leading candidate-in groups. He may with permission leave the house for personal reasons or business and may occasionally spend an evening out. He has begun to assume authority not only over others within the house, but the even more difficult task over self in the world at large. After he is observed to be functioning at a mature level, he may be sponsored for the candidacy-out or the second stage of re-entry. He must affirmatively answer the question: "Will I leave the protective shelter of Odyssey House for the community at large?"

The Inquiry-Out is a meeting before his own peer group, the one above, and the staff. Here, the proposed candidate-out discusses his future plans, presents a reintegration program, and is questioned in detail as to the realities of the outside world in relation to himself. He must consider and choose alternatives in the social and work areas. If the plan is considered complete and realistic, he is voted a candidate-out. At this level he may begin to put it into effect.

In the period of the candidacy-out, the resident acts upon and effects his reintegration plan. He may start school or formal vocational training. He must have obtained a High School Equivalency diploma as a level IV if he is not a high school graduate. He must hold employment outside of the field of drug addiction. He spends increasing time with his family, spending overnights or weekends with them. He may marry or divorce during this period. He must answer the question: "Will I succeed?" in the affirmative.

The candidate-out lives outside the program as an independent, functioning, useful citizen. He is salaried and a taxpayer. If he is employed at Odyssey House, his involvement with the program becomes more intense and demanding. If he works in other fields, his contact with Odyssey House is limited to weekly candidate-out groups in the evening which are geared by a physician or the Director of the Program. He continues to give up urine on a regular (but unscheduled) basis.

The last challenge to the candidate-out is the Probe-Out, which constitutes discharge to outpatient status.

This is the most important evaluation in the program because once the candidate-out becomes an outpatient, he is considered independent of the program except for occasional urinanalysis. The only therapy requirement will be a periodic group session, for approximately two or three years after discharge.

In about 30 percent of the residents, problems of a neurotic nature are unmasked when the sociopathic behavior patterns are lifted. Just prior to or at the time of re-entry, if one of these patients requests, he will be referred to individual therapy, but this must be in addition to the continuing group work. Individual work is permissible and desirable at this time. These patients now have the prerequisite anxiety to make them amenable to therapy, they can form the necessary transference relationships, and they can control their behavior sufficiently to keep appointments. Once salaried, they will independently negotiate on a fee-for-service basis with the treating psychiatrist.

The last phase needs no further discussion as the participant, except for the reservations listed above, functions as any other member of society. He has become a full-functioning, independent, constructive member of society. Most have chosen lives independent of their past drug usage; others have chosen employment within the field of drug addiction and prevention.

Since most of Odyssey patients are under no external pressure to completing the treatment process, many decide to leave Odyssey prior to graduation. Nevertheless, even those patients who do not complete the treatment program are impressively influenced. Follow-up studies have shown that 75 percent of the former patients go on to lead drug free, crime free, and productively employed lives. Of the many who do graduate the program, success is significantly higher, including those who go on to pursue careers in health care, medicine, law, finance and business.

The concept under which the community flourishes has been expressed in the following ways by its residents:

(1)   Positive growth occurs in the soil of self-knowledge which is best seen in the mirror of peer group interaction.

(2)   We see ourselves best in the eye of a brother. Therefore, the brother must open his eyes and speak honestly what he sees.

(3)   The basic concept of our program is continual open confrontation with the reality of ourselves, our peers, and our environment.

(4)   By open confrontation, and the experience of the concern of others for me, for the first time in my life, I have learned first to trust and then to cope positively. First I coped a little, now big.

(5)   And finally, it is the rule of three. First by doing, I proved that it can be done. The second doing followed with ease, and the third slipped by unnoticed. I had a habit of living.

21

Research Design, Drug Use, and Deaths: Cross Study Comparisons

DON C. DES JARLAIS

The issue of appropriate research designs for studying heroin use and treatment for heroin addiction is one of the more problematic in the field. The true experiment, with random assignment of subjects to treatment versus no treatment is generally considered the surest path to valid knowledge in both medicine and social science (Campbell and Stanley, 1963, the classic statement of the virtues of experimental design). With respect to the treatment of heroin addiction, there is a generally held belief that the patients' life situations have been rapidly deteriorating just prior to beginning treatment, and thus might be expected to improve over time even if treatment is not provided.

Despite the apparent desirability of using randomized experiments to assess treatment for heroin addiction there are a host of difficulties in doing so. Dole and Singer (1979) have discussed these ethical, practical, and theoretical problems in detail. An illustrative case is the one study in which random assignment was attempted, (Bale et al, 1978) but patients migrated away from the assigned treatment to the treatments of their choice. Thus what had started as a true randomized assignment study became confounded with patient self-selection—acceptance of the treatments assigned.

In view of the great difficulties in doing true experiments in the treatment of chronic heroin addiction, it becomes important to determine whether similar substantive findings are obtained with a variety of research designs. This paper will examine substantive results from three studies of chronic heroin addicts that differed greatly with respect to research design issues. The substantive areas to be considered are drug use and deaths. The three studies to be examined are a treatment follow-up study of methadone maintenance patients in New York City (Des Jarlais et al, 1981; Dole and Joseph, 1979), a true randomized experiment of methadone treatment in Sweden (Gunne, 1981) and an oral history study of elderly narcotic users (Courtwright, Joseph and Des Jarlais, in press).

TECHNICAL DIFFERENCES AMONG THE STUDIES

The research designs are undoubtedly the greatest difference among the studies. The Swedish study used a classic experimental design with subjects who applied for treatment being randomly assigned to either methadone maintenance treatment or to no treatment. The design was maintained over time, with the no treatment group not receiving any formal treatment. Comparisons were thus made between those who did not receive treatment with those who received continuous methadone maintenance treatment. The follow-up of the New York City study used a longitudinal design. Comparisons were made of the pre-treatment, during treatment and post-treatment periods for the same subjects. The oral history study involved life history interviews with a group of elderly (fifty-five years or older) narcotic users. To the extent that comparisons were made, they were between the subjects' behavior and the reported behavior of other narcotic users known to the subjects. The three studies can easily be ranked on a scale of "methodological rigor" from true experiment to pre-experimental (Campbell and Stanley, 1963).

The studies varied in other important aspects. The Swedish study had a relatively small sample size—seventeen in the experiment treatment group and seventeen in the control group. The New York follow-up study, in contrast, had a sample size of 1,500. The oral history study had an intermediate sample size of 50.

The social context in which the subjects lived varied in the three studies. Sweden is a socially homogenous country, in which the heroin addiction problem is relatively new. The New York City follow-up study had as its context the city that has been called "the heroin capital of the world." The study covered a time period (roughly from 1966 to 1975) when the city saw the highest incidence of heroin use in its history. The oral history study was also primarily based in New York City (all subjects were recruited while living in New York) but spans the time period from the 1920s to the present. It thus covers the wide variations in public policy, treatment availability, and heroin availability that have existed in New York City over the last 60 years.

There are several similarities among the studies that should also be noted. First, all three studies included only subjects who had applied for treatment at least once in their lives. They did not include persons who only experimented with heroin or who managed to successfully self-treat problems associated with heroin use. Second, all studies covered relatively long periods of time. From a minimum of two years in the Swedish study to over sixty years in the oral history study. Finally, all three studies include periods in which the subjects lived in their "natural" communities. They were not confined to residential treatment settings or hospitals for the duration of the study. These similarities among the studies lead to some expectation of similarities in the substantive findings, and also serve to distinguish these three studies from other studies using the same research designs but different subjects, shorter time periods or more restricted settings.

The methodological differences among the studies are still sufficiently great that different findings could be easily attributed to the differences in methods. Two types of substantive findings will be examined across the three studies—drug use and deaths.

DRUG USE

The fundamental question in assessing the effectiveness of treatment for heroin addiction is whether the declines in heroin use that are typically seen during treatment (and to a lesser extent after treatment) "caused" by treatment, or would they have occurred without treatment being provided. The Swedish study, through the use of a random assignment control group, provides the easiest to interpret answer to this question. Heroin use in the methadone maintenance treatment group declined to essentially zero. Heroin use in the untreated group remained very high—twelve subjects were using heroin at the time of follow-up, two were in prison, two had died, and only one had managed to become abstinent without formal treatment (or incarceration).

In the New York City follow-up study, the question of the effectiveness of treatment in reducing heroin use is answered by comparisons of three different time periods for the same subjects: prior to, during, and after treatment. Figure 1 shows the heroin use for 528 subjects in this study during the study period and for whom complete drug histories were obtained. There is a clear suppression of heroin use during treatment with a frequent return to heroin use after treatment.

The drop in heroin use from the prior to the during treatment periods is too large to be plausibily attributed to other factors than the provision of methadone treatment. Similarly, the return to heroin use after treatment is too large not to be associated with the cessation of treatment.

The oral history study does not directly address the question of the impact of treatment on illicit heroin use. It does, however, cover a period from the 1920s to the 1960s when there was very little treatment available

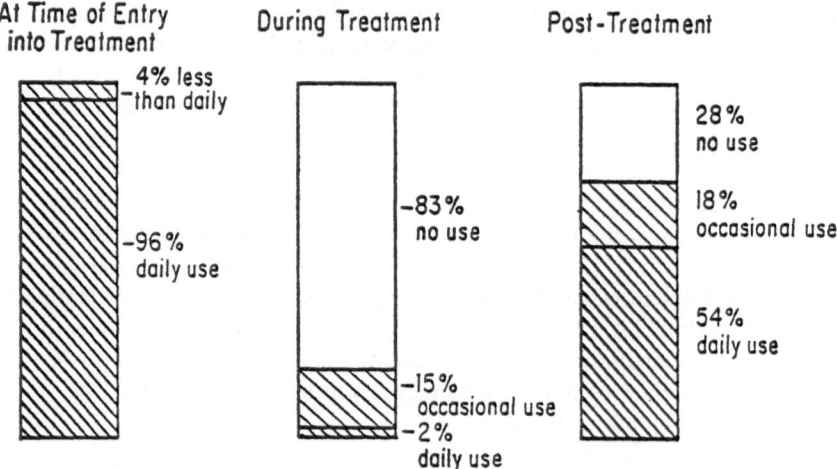

Fig. 1. Incidence of illicit narcotic use before, during and after methadone maintenance treatment (528 subjects).

for heroin addiction. Thus the heroin use of during this period can be considered an estimate of heroin use in the absence of public treatment, for this admittedly atypical group of heroin users. In describing their use of narcotics, the oral history subjects do not mention frequent or long periods of abstinence. Instead they describe their ability to obtain an almost continuous supply of narcotics, even during periods such as World War II, when the illicit supply was probably at its lowest point during the century. These subjects had what seem to be unusually good connections for obtaining narcotics in the illicit market, as well as a well honed ability to obtain narcotic prescriptions from private physicians.

When discussing the specifics of their use of narcotics, these subjects mention a controlled style of use, even though they were using on at least a daily basis. They emphasize that they would use their "regular" amount, that they "were not greedy," and did go on binges where they would consume all of the narcotics that they could obtain.

The oral history subjects are clearly an atypical group of narcotic users, but they do provide evidence against the hypothesis that narcotic addiction will decline in the absence of formal treatment (Snow, 1973; and Waldorf, in press) for evidence in support of such a hypothesis. The inference from the oral history study is thus consistent with the Swedish and the New York City methadone studies: illicit narcotic use will continue at very high levels in the absence of formal treatment among persons who have established a chronic pattern of heroin use.

DEATHS

Drug related deaths may be considered the ultimate form of substance abuse. From their different methodological perspectives, the studies discussed here provide similar insights into the relationships between heroin use and death. The Swedish study found that none of the persons admitted to methadone maintenance dies within the two year follow-up period, while two of the seventeen persons who were randomly denied methadone treatment died, for a death rate of six percent per year. This difference in death rates can only be considered suggestive, however, because of the small sample size.

A major advantage of large scale longitudinal studies is that they can provide stable estimates of death rates and estimates of risk factors. Table 1 presents death rates and causes of death for the New York City study. The during treatment death rate is 1.5 percent per year, while the post-treatment rate rises to 3.5 percent per year. The major difference in the causes of deaths is the opiate related deaths. The preponderance of these opiate related deaths came shortly after the subjects had terminated from methadone maintenance treatment. They had usually detoxified as part of termination and presumably had not developed sufficient tolerance to counteract the varying quality of illicitly obtained narcotics. The size of the sample in the New York City methadone follow-up study provides statistical confirmation

Table 1. Numbers of Deaths and Death Rates by Treatment Status and Cause of Death

| Cause of Death | During Maintenance | | After Maintenance | |
	N	Rate per 1,000 Person– Years	N	Rate per 1,000 Person– Years
Drug Related	37	6.0	56	24.0
Total Opiates	2	0.3	36	15.3
Opiates Only	2	0.3	19	8.1
with Alcohol	0	0	15	6.4
with Nonopiates	0	0	2	0.9
Alcohol	31	5.1	17	7.2
Nonopiates	4	0.7	3	1.3
Violence	15	2.5	14	6.0
Accident	5	0.8	1	0.4
Unknown	8	1.3	6	2.6
Medical	28	4.6	6	2.6
Total	93	15.2	83	35.3

of the treatment lowered death rates that were suggested by the random assignment Swedish study. It also provides the most probable reason for the excess deaths in the non-treatment period.

Since all subjects in the oral history study were alive at the time of interview, and there has not yet been sufficient follow-up to note death rates, the only evidence from this study about drug related deaths is again indirect. In some ways this study may provide the most interesting insights into the relationships between heroin use and death. Clearly the subjects of this study lived well beyond the normal life span for heroin addicts. A major focus of the study is to determine the reasons for this unexpected longevity. The analysis of the reasons for longevity is not yet completed, but two of the reasons that the subjects give for their longevity have already been noted—their ability to obtain regular supplies of narcotics and their self-regulated use of narcotics. The two other reasons that are frequently given by the subjects are their ability to minimize their involvement in the "street life" and the scrupulous care they took to insure the cleanliness of the needles they used for injecting narcotics.

CONCLUSION

The three studies briefly discussed here had similar subject populations—persons who had become chronically addicted to narcotics. Despite the great differences in the methodologies used in the three studies, they all provide strong support for the hypotheses that maintenance treatment both greatly reduces illicit narcotic use and death rates for these persons.

At a deeper level of analysis, the three studies all point to the desirability, and perhaps the inevitability, of narcotic maintenance treatment once illicit narcotic use has become established within a society. If narcotic maintenance treatment is not publicly provided within such a society, there will be a small group of chronic narcotic users who managed to create their own private maintenance programs. Their narcotic use will be characterized by a relatively continuous use of narcotics, in relatively carefully regulated dosages, and with great concern for hygiene. These persons will also seek to avoid the dangerous street subculture that surrounds much of illicit narcotic use. The creation of these self-maintenance programs is testimony to both the intractibility of narcotic use among such individuals, and, given their narcotic addiction, a remarkable set of coping skills.

If narcotic maintenance treatment programs are publicly provided, then more suitable substances for the most suitable narcotics for maintenance can be readily utilized, hygienic conditions much more easily achieved, and alternatives to involvement in the street subculture encouraged for much greater numbers of chronic narcotic users. Clearly, not all persons who use illicit narcotics nor even all persons who have become addicted for lengthy periods of time, are suitable candidates for narcotic maintenance treatment. But for the sizable percentage of illicit narcotic users who do need maintenance treatment, the greater availability of publicly provided maintenance will be not only a matter of reducing illicit drug use and involvement in the street subcultures, but also, literally, a matter of life and death.

REFERENCES

Bale R, Van Stone WW, Englesing TJJ and Zarcone VP: Preliminary 2-year follow-up results from a randomized comparison of methadone maintenance and therapeutic communities. In: Smith DE, Anderson SM, Buxton M, Gottlieb N, Harvey W and Chung T (eds) *A Multi-Cultural View of Drug Abuse.* Cambridge, Mass.: Schenkman, 1978

Campbell DT and Stanley JC: *Experimental and Quasi-Experimental Design for Research.* Chicago: Rand-McNally, 1963

Courtwright D, Joseph H and Des Jarlais DC: Oral histories of elderly methadone patients. *Journal of Oral History* (in press)

Des Jarlais DC, Joseph H and Dole VP: Long term outcomes after termination from methadone maintenance treatment. *Ann NY Acad Sci* 362:231–238, 1981

Dole VP and Joseph H: Long term consequences of methadone maintenance treatment. Final report to National Institute of Drug Abuse, contract 5H81DA01778-02, 1979

Dole VP and Singer B: On the evaluation of treatments for narcotic addiction. *Journal of Drug Issues* 205–211, Spring 1979

Gunne L: The Swedish methadone maintenance treatment experience. *Drug Alc Dep* 1981

Snow M: Maturing out of narcotic addiction in New York City. *International Journal of the Addictions* 8:921–938, 1973

Waldorf D: Natural recovery from opiate addiction: Some social psychological processes of untreated recovery. *Journal of Drug Issues* (in press)

Index